Bad Habits, Hard Choices

PERSPECTIVES

Series editor: Diane Coyle

Bad Habits, Hard Choices

Using the Tax System to
Make Us Healthier

David Fell

LONDON PUBLISHING PARTNERSHIP

Published by London Publishing Partnership
www.londonpublishingpartnership.co.uk

Published in association with
Enlightenment Economics
www.enlightenmenteconomics.com

ISBN: 978-1-907994-50-0 (pbk)

A catalogue record for this book is
available from the British Library

This book has been composed in Candara

Copy-edited and typeset by
T&T Productions Ltd, London
www.tandtproductions.com

Cover art by Kate Prentice

Printed by Page Bros, Norwich

Contents

CONTENTS

Preface

In many ways this book is a continuation of what I now realize is a lifelong obsession with choice: what it is, how it works and why we make the choices that we do. It's an obsession that is personal, professional, political and philosophical, as I think this book illustrates.

Bad habits

My professional research has covered a wide range of social and environmental choices that we as individuals and as a society make. It is, however, the choices we make about food that have been the most pronounced focus of my work over the past couple of decades. My obsession hinges, I think, on the scale of the mismatch between the choices we say we want to make and the choices we actually make. We all want to be healthy; but we eat and drink in ways that make us ill.

So in this book I've taken the opportunity to step back from the specifics of food waste, animal welfare, use-by dates and air miles to go as deep as I can into the whys and wherefores of the choices we make about food.

I draw on insights from behavioural economics, social psychology and linguistics to suggest that the narratives of modern marketing have been comprehensively internalized by the majority of the population. These narratives frame some choices as 'good' and some as 'bad'.

The choices we make as consumers are frequently good for capitalism and bad for us. Over-buying and over-eating are conspicuous examples. The persistence of these bad habits, I argue, is the outcome of the mismatch in power between corporatized marketing, on the one hand, and frail and fallible individuals, on the other. Expecting individuals each to overcome their bad habits is misguided. An effective solution needs to redress the power imbalance and has therefore to be of significant institutional scale.

Hard choices

Introducing the notion of 'commitment strategies' developed by the Nobel-winning economist Thomas Schelling, and considering also the techniques of deliberative democracy, I then explain and illustrate how power imbalances can be redressed in ways that are inclusive, fair, adaptable and resilient.

I go on to suggest that a suitably configured 'socially determined commitment strategy' has the potential to counteract the power of modern marketing and to frame a new narrative in which healthy eating is both straightforward and – crucially – affordable.

Four steps

I set out a concrete proposition for how such a strategy could be introduced. I propose that negative VAT should be charged on healthy foods and high VAT should be charged on unhealthy foods. I set out a four-step process to implement this new regime, each step of which depends on mechanisms that have already been used by government.

It is, I acknowledge, a bold proposition, and one that certainly goes far beyond the idea of a sugar tax or a fat tax. Indeed, in the final chapter I speculate on whether the basic idea could be extended to address an even wider range of social and environmental ills.

Such speculation may be misplaced at this early stage, but it is perhaps consistent with the obsession that seems to have propelled this book into existence; and it is, in the end, no more than a choice I happen to have made.

Acknowledgements

To Diane, Richard and Sam; James and Alex; Paul, Samantha, Robin, Lilian, Tim, Jayne, Rachel, Martin, Alice, David, Xristina and Inge; and everyone at Brook Lyndhurst – thank you. You all helped, or hindered constructively, and I am grateful.

Chapter 1

Let's go shopping

I'm all lost in the supermarket

— *The Clash*

Just like millions of other people, last week I went
shopping. Nothing special: a trip to the supermarket. I
bought my usual groceries, enough for the week's meals.
I bought a couple of bottles of wine, too. I'm lucky: I earn
just enough not to pay too much attention to the prices.
I put the things I wanted in the trolley, picking up a few
things I hadn't intended to buy, but comfortable that I
was avoiding anything exorbitantly expensive.

Generally I try to buy organic or Fairtrade or locally
produced food if I can, but I don't try all that hard. If
there's an attractive bargain, or the price of the eth-
ical alternative seems too high, I'll edit my choices
accordingly. Most of the time – and this was certainly the
case last week – I rely on my usual brands. I always buy
Lavazza coffee, for example. I'm not sure why: there are

dozens of types of coffee on the shelf, and I've tried just a handful.

At the till, just like millions of other people, I did my part of the deal – unloading and then reloading my trolley – before handing over my plastic. I typed my four memorable digits into the little black rectangle, glanced at the bill and headed out of the shop.

I'd arranged to meet a good friend for a drink that same day, so once I'd dumped all the shopping into the cupboards and the fridge at home I set off in my car. I stopped at the petrol station, stocked up on fuel, chocolate and – ahem – cigarettes, and drove the thirty-odd miles to Hertfordshire. It wasn't a particularly long evening: we ate a light meal, had a couple of drinks, two coffees, and then I headed home.

My bill in the supermarket was £78.24. At the petrol station I spent £64.97 on fuel, £3 on chocolate and £9.69 on cigarettes. In the evening I spent £12.50 on my meal, £8.40 on two pints of beer and £4.60 on two cups of coffee. All told, £181.40.

In my book, that's quite a steep day. I know that the groceries and the petrol will last me a few days, but even so – nearly two hundred pounds!

The real shocker, though, is that without knowing I was doing so I had paid out £43.20 in tax.

My monthly salary slip tells me exactly how much tax I've paid; why not the slip at the checkout? This seems odd. It can't be that hard, surely, to display how much of the price of each item on the shelf is tax? Then, if I wanted, I could make different choices and avoid paying that tax.

And why am I paying taxes on some of the items and not others? Is it an untrustworthy government fleecing me yet again? Or are they trying to discourage me from driving and smoking and drinking (and if it is that, why not make it clearer)? Or perhaps it's just a ridiculous mess: a porridge of out-of-date ideas and priorities, as uncomfortable and daunting for the officials, politicians and statisticians as it is opaque, confusing and unfair for the rest of us. Maybe it's all of the above?

This book is about how to sort this mess out – not for the sake of it, but to show how we could use something boring like tax to do really exciting things like help people lose weight and live well, and perhaps even help to save the planet.

Our VAT system – in fact, our entire edifice of 'consumer-facing taxes' – is both damaging and stupid. It arrived in the UK when we joined the European Community in 1973, a time so unimaginably distant it is difficult even to begin describing how different it was. It is not simply that there were no mobile phones or computers or barcodes; the entire universe of 'choices' available to the consumer – what to buy, where to buy, when to buy – had barely evolved since World War II. Yet the basic structure and rules of the VAT system in 2015 are unchanged since that era of rotary dial phones, type-writers, flares and platform boots.

It's time for SmartVAT. It's time to haul it into the twenty-first century and make use of the barcodes and the IT, as well as all the insights we now have about shopping and consumption and human behaviour. And if we're going to go to the trouble of making it smart, we might just as well make it *really* smart. Let's see if we can actually *reduce* the price of the things we know are good – things that keep us healthy, for example, or things that help the environment, or things that help the weakest and most vulnerable people live a decent life – and *increase* the price, by quite a lot, of the things that cause harm.

Tax, it has to be said, can seem pretty dull. But so are seat belts, washing your hands before eating and lots of other everyday things. Almost everyone managed to agree that it was just plain sensible to wear a seat belt; and we all know that basic hygiene is common sense. And, every day, just like millions of other people, we navigate our way among dozens or hundreds or even thousands of complete strangers as we go about our daily lives; and generally we are cooperative and nice to one another. Imagine if we insert into that everyday miracle of cooperation a smart tax system that makes us smart consumers.

The rest of this book explains why it is such good sense for the government to change the way it taxes the products we buy every day, not least because we are human beings rather than the mythical 'rational agents' of economic theory. We do not have time to calculate the pros and cons of every choice, but instead use rules of thumb, or are persuaded by the stories told about 'brands' – or we just give in to temptation. We are manipulated by businesses that make big profits from selling us unhealthy and damaging products.

This book also explains *how* to bring about the transition to SmartVAT. It is a very practical proposal whose four elements are already used in other contexts. The biggest step will be the first: believing that there *is* a way of committing ourselves to healthier choices, in a fairer system, that will raise at least as much money for the Treasury as is now raised.

Dull? Sounds terrific to me.

Chapter 2

The taxes we pay

If you drive a car, I'll tax the street
If you try to sit, I'll tax your seat
If you get too cold I'll tax the heat
If you take a walk, I'll tax your feet
— *George Harrison*

Consumers in Britain pay a curious mix of taxes when they spend their money. Most obviously, they pay value added tax, or VAT, on all the things they buy. Except that VAT *isn't* charged on everything: it isn't charged on books or children's clothes, for example. It isn't charged on food, either. Except when it is. Somewhere, hidden on a transparent government website,[1] there is a mighty list of all the exceptions – you pay VAT on ice cream, for example, but not on frozen yoghurt; you don't pay VAT on a flapjack, but you do if you buy a cereal bar.

VAT came into being back in the early 1970s as a condition of joining the European Community (as it was then). It replaced taxes such as purchase tax and luxury goods tax and considerable effort went into designing the new tax in a way that the government of the time thought was fair. A key tenet of fairness was that certain basic items – such as food, books and children's clothes – should not be taxed. However, it was also considered fair that certain not-so-basic items should *not* be tax free; after all, only wealthy people bought these not-so-basic items, and at the time that VAT was introduced the top income tax rate being paid by the country's wealthiest people was – take a deep breath – 83%.

So wise and caring officials and statisticians carefully looked through the catalogue of all the various food products available on the nation's shelves and allocated them to one of two lists: one list for food items that anyone might buy and another for foods bought only by the rich.

And they did it again the next year, too, because quite a number of new products became available, all of which needed to be classified.

And then again the next year, and the next year, and the year after that.

As you can imagine, the lists became quite long. Dauntingly long, in fact. So long that the thought of, say, having a bit of a rethink about which items were on which list, or how many lists there were, or whether the original basis for the lists even made sense anymore... Well, such thoughts were simply unthinkable: it would take too much time, too much effort and – let's face it – it would cause too much political trouble.

In any case, as successive governments discovered, the great British public seemed not to notice VAT most of the time, and this invisible tax consistently delivered a very useful chunk of money to the Treasury.[2] There was little incentive to make any big changes and some very good reasons for leaving well alone.

But of course VAT is not the only tax surreptitiously confronting the British consumer. Much more high profile, for example, are the taxes on alcohol and tobacco. These taxes get their own special name – 'duty' – and they are usually part of an annual political ritual in which they are either dramatically increased or kept the same by a Chancellor of the Exchequer whenever he (so far it's always been a he) performs a Budget. These taxes, too, are opaque at the point of sale; and, like VAT, they have a rationale that becomes more and more curious the closer you look.

Tobacco tax, for starters, has been increasing relentlessly for decades and is currently well above 100%. (Actually, it varies, because part of the tax is a fixed sum of money – £3.79[3] – so the cheaper your cigarettes, the higher the rate of tax you pay.) This is almost universally seen as a 'good thing'. Smoking is bad for one's health, so it has become accepted that government discourages us from smoking by increasing the price of cigarettes. This is in turn some pretty basic economics: in general, the more costly a thing is, the less of it we buy.

The *rate* at which government has increased tobacco duty is perhaps more interesting. On the one hand, the money raised from taxing tobacco was and remains non-trivial,[4] and no government would wish to see too much of that revenue disappear too suddenly. On the other hand, people are at liberty to smoke if they wish, and to punish or be seen to punish too large a group of people simply on the grounds of a choice they are making would run political risks. So a balancing act is perpetually called for.

And, of course, there's a third hand that we mustn't forget: the tobacco industry, which for decades was big and strong and intimidating and most certainly needed to be considered if you, the lowly Chancellor of the Exchequer, were thinking about annoying them by causing their sales (and revenue and profit) to decline. The balancing act is very precarious indeed.

A similar balancing act has applied in the case of alcohol taxes. The companies that manufacture alcohol are big and strong and intimidating; the British people have a right to drink as much alcohol as they like, even if it's bad for them; and government raises a lot of money by taxing alcohol.[2] Alcohol is not as straightforward as tobacco, though, because there are lots of different types of alcoholic drink – all with differing strengths, all drunk by different groups of people in society and made by businesses of differing degrees of scariness.

Like VAT, alcohol duties are not made apparent when you buy your drink; and it may therefore be something of a shock to discover that the amount of tax you pay depends on a whole range of arbitrary boundaries. Hand the barman £3 or £4 for a pint of relatively weak ale and you pay a paltry 11 pence in tax. Hand the barman the same amount of money for the adjacent ale, just a little stronger, and you pay 47 pence in tax. Something similar applies if your tipple is cider or wine (and whether it fizzes or not makes a difference to how much tax you pay, too).

Awareness of the health and social costs associated with alcohol consumption has lagged awareness of tobacco's ill effects, and it is only within the past decade or so that the idea of using taxes to limit our consumption has been aired in public. Minimum unit pricing,[5] for example, has been suggested as a way in which all alcohol could be taxed on a consistent (if not necessarily fair) basis – and resistance to this idea has come from predictable voices and with predictable outrage.

The same kind of outrage – a mix of menaces from scary businesses, loud newspapers and indignant citizens – will be familiar with regard to petrol, another area where opaque taxes are paid by the customer. Fuel prices vary like topsy because of the international oil price, as we know, but the average British consumer is currently paying in the region of 135% tax on their fuel.

Yes, you read that correctly. (Imagine if it was clearly advertised at the point of sale.)

Once upon a time, and not so long ago, the fuel duty escalator[6] represented an intention to increase the tax on petrol and other fuels at a steady rate, specifically to encourage us (the great British car-borne consumer) to use less fuel, which would in turn help reduce our carbon dioxide emissions, in turn helping save the planet. Here we see something similar to the situation with alcohol and tobacco: microeconomics teaches us that, as the price of a good rises, demand falls. The more expensive a thing is, the less of it you buy.

Well, up to a point. And it is a point at which economics brings in two other ideas: 'other things being equal' and 'elasticity'. The idea of 'other things being equal' is simply the elimination of all other factors that could be influencing your choice: as the price of, say, honey goes up, the amount you buy goes down – but only if nothing else changes. You might, for example, occasionally buy jam instead of honey, so if honey becomes more expensive, you might simply switch to jam – unless, of course, the price of jam has *also* increased. Ditto peanut butter, Marmite and so on. To eliminate all these possible complications, economists deploy the phrase 'other things being equal'.

More important, however, is the notion of 'elasticity'. It concerns the responsiveness of the amount you buy to a price change. If the amount you buy changes relatively little in response to a price change (whether the price goes up or down), then your demand is deemed to be 'inelastic'; whereas if it changes a lot, it is 'elastic'.

By and large, if you (and everyone else) 'need' a product – that is, the more that it is a basic requirement of modern life as opposed to a frippery – the more inelastic is demand. This is reinforced still further if there are few alternatives available. So take something like bread, the price of which depends largely on the price of wheat, an everyday staple of British diets: if the price goes up, the scope for switching to something else is limited; and the scope for not having bread is also pretty limited. We could reasonably expect the demand for bread to be inelastic.

Honey, on the other hand, is much less of a staple, and it is a product for which a number of alternatives exist: demand is likely to be more elastic for honey than for bread.

What about petrol? Or alcohol? Or tobacco?

The answer matters very much to government, and most especially the Treasury. If demand is relatively *inelastic*, then the amount we buy isn't likely to fall too much if the price goes up, so an increase in tax could be expected to have relatively little impact on the total amount we buy. That would in turn mean that tax revenue would go up, manufacturers wouldn't suffer and go on to cause the government headaches, and, so long as we consumers can absorb the increase, we would tend not to complain. But if we can't absorb it – if it just hurts too much (as started to happen in response to the fuel duty escalator) – our complaints can become loud and, eventually, politically significant.*

Intriguingly, no one really knows for sure what the various elasticities are since, in the real world, things are very much *not* equal; and things are always changing. So a degree of judgment rather than mathematics is always involved, and this in turn means that it's always at least as much about politics as it is about economics.

Or perhaps there's a more precise way of putting that: since, in actual fact, it is the innumerable choices of perfectly ordinary human beings that comprise these elasticities, then we are very clearly in the realm of human behaviour – which means we could draw on social psychology, or sociology, or law, or philosophy, or even faith or fiction to understand what is going on. No wonder it's complicated.

---

* Here is another important feature of elasticity. It is relatively straightforward to switch from honey to jam, but it is not so easy to change the amount of fuel you use, particularly if most of your mileage comes from regularly driving to and from work. One obvious option is to choose a more fuel-efficient car when you come to replace your vehicle, and you may well do so in response to the higher cost of fuel; but this response happens, clearly, over a different kind of time-frame.

Perhaps tired of this complexity, the people now known as behavioural economists set about conducting experiments. Rather than merely pontificating or theorizing or extrapolating, they began devising tests intended to explore what people actually *do* when confronted with this or that choice. It's a moot point precisely when these experiments started but – for the purposes of this particular book at least – the key moment may well have been when Daniel Kahneman won the Nobel Memorial Prize in Economic Sciences in 2002. Kahneman was not only one of the pioneers of these experiments, he was the first non-economist to win the Nobel Prize in Economics. It was, and remains, a key sign that some of the most basic assumptions that economics has long made about human behaviour are simply wrong.

I'll come back to that later. In the meantime, Kahneman's work – alongside that of many more famous and less famous others – has secured a foothold in the circles where such things as VAT are known as policy instruments. Beginning a decade or so ago, in particular following the publishing success of *Nudge*,[7] a variety of government departments began their own experiments, looking at something called behaviour change. Apart from asking nicely, governments only really have two policy instruments at their disposal: fiscal measures (i.e. money) and regulatory measures (i.e. laws).*

---

* Note also that the *threat* of new laws or regulations is in the mix (and often lurks behind the 'asking nicely').

Tobacco provides the perfect illustration: they ask us nicely to smoke less, by advertising what it does to our lungs or our babies; they increase the price (a fiscal measure); and they ban smoking in public places (a regulatory measure).

Behaviour change is, potentially, a new tool in the box. The experiments conducted by Kahneman and others have progressively revealed a whole bunch of human behaviours that are reasonably predictable and, irrespective of your theoretical or political or philosophical perspective, are nevertheless 'true'. Humans have defaults, for example: which means, crudely, that we tend to go along with how things are rather than make the effort of changing. One of the best illustrations concerns organ donation: the default in Britain is 'no thanks'. It requires a specific effort by an individual to register as an organ donor and, as a result, not enough people ever register. In a number of continental European countries – including Belgium, France and Poland – the default is 'yes please'. No one is *obliged* to offer their organs for transplant in the event of their death, but in these countries an individual has to make a specific effort to *de*-register. The number of organ donors is incomparably higher in these countries than in the UK.[8]

This intervention involved neither a regulatory change nor a fiscal change, but it was extremely effective. It was also cheap.

So here we have a new way in which government might try to achieve its objectives: if regulation is too unpalatable and taxes just annoy everyone, let's see if there's some subtle change we could make in the cues or the defaults or the guidance or the wording or whatever that would have the effect we're after.

At this point I'm hoping at least a bit of you is thinking: hang on a minute, that sounds like I'm being manipulated by the government – which doesn't sound at all fair.

To which my answers are: yes, you are being manipulated; and no, it's not fair. But that's not the interesting part of the story. The interesting part is that not only are big companies – the people who want to sell you a new phone, a new holiday destination, a new culinary opportunity – performing exactly these tricks on each and every one of us every single day, they are also deploying a simply staggering array of these techniques, all of the time. They have been doing it for so long, and have become so good at it, that we no longer even notice.

Is *that* fair?

In the case of these big corporations, it is at least possible to acknowledge something of the form, 'well, they would do that, wouldn't they?' After all, they exist to sell us whatever it is they make (it's hardly complicated), so it's inevitable that they'd put a lot of effort into selling us stuff, even if – perhaps *especially* if – we didn't really want it.

But governments? Have we really authorized them to manipulate us? Or to hide these taxes that we're paying?

And how come they're taxing the things we buy anyway? The very economic theory that the world's economic powerhouses believe in actually suggests there shouldn't be any of these taxes at all.

Chapter 3

The informed consumer?

> It is in the spirit of the age to believe that any fact, no matter how suspect, is superior to any imaginative exercise, no matter how true.
>
> — *Gore Vidal*

The men and women responsible for deciding how much tax we pay on our beer and our petrol and our sweets work in the same department of government as the people responsible for overall economic policy. These people – economists – are custodians of a theory that they use to devise economic policy.* This theory – which states, roughly, that free and competitive markets always deliver the best possible outcomes, and which

---

* Full disclosure: the author studied economics to degree level and for many years had the word 'economist' in his job title. Curiously – or perhaps not – there is no professional body for economists; so unlike, say, doctors or lawyers or architects, there is no particular set of qualifications required to be an economist. Quite why anyone might want to call themselves an economist is a mystery, but anyone could, if they wanted to. As it happens, I now increasingly describe myself as a 'recovering economist'.

from here onwards I shall call simply the Theory – has achieved extraordinary power and status in recent decades: it lies at the heart of the belief system of not just the UK Treasury, but of all the major economic institutions of the world – the European Commission, the International Monetary Fund, the US government, the World Bank.

This same belief system also characterizes the finance and economics teams of all the other economic powerhouses of the world: the banks, the investment houses, the private equity businesses, the multinational corporations. (Perhaps this is not surprising: these two communities – the 'markets' and the 'regulators' – deal only with each other, so they need to speak the same language.)

It is a virtual requirement of employment in any of these institutions that an individual must profess wholehearted belief in the Theory and its associated tenets. To ensure appropriate immersion in the relevant beliefs, the world's leading educational establishments compete with each other to supply a steady stream of suitably processed young economists to these various institutions.

Roughly speaking, the theory that dominates the economic policies of the UK, the EU, North America and pretty much everywhere else requires its adherents to believe three things.

- First, that the 'best' possible outcomes will come about when markets operate 'efficiently'.
- Second, this efficiency can be achieved by ensuring effective competition between businesses (by removing impediments to the ability of businesses to do whatever it is they do).
- And third, that consumers have the information necessary to make effective choices between the goods and services offered by the businesses competing for their custom.

The last of these is the requirement for what is called the 'informed consumer'. It's a simple and alluring idea: if we consumers have all the information we need, we can choose confidently between the available options; and the businesses providing the goods or services that best meet our needs (or wants) will thrive, while those that fail to do so have a simple Darwinian choice: adapt or die.

The impact of the belief is ubiquitous: it is why our electrical products have energy labels, so we can choose how much energy we want our fridges and ovens to consume; it is why our cars have official fuel consumption figures, so we can choose the level of emissions we want; it is why the labels on our food have details of all the ingredients and nutritional values and significance to our average daily requirements and so forth, so we can choose what to eat.

The trouble is that while this 'informed consumer' might be fine in theory, in practice he or she does not exist.

In theory, individual human beings make rational decisions about how much time they wish to invest in gathering information before making a purchase, and they are therefore optimally informed. Add up all of the millions and millions of consumers and the result is a market in which information is being used efficiently, so the economic outcomes must be efficient and – lo! – we have the Theory, capital T.

In practice, however, the 'informed consumer' is the conjoined twin of the 'rational economic (hu)man'. These myths, just like all myths, played a vital role when no better explanation of the world was available. But, just as the idea of 'rational economic (hu)man' has been progressively discredited in recent years – not least by the behavioural experiments that were briefly discussed above – so too must go the idea of the informed consumer. It might be uncomfortable in the corridors and bunkers where the high priests and acolytes of the Theory reside; and uncomfortable, too, for the rest of us, not least because a fully-fledged replacement for the Theory does not yet exist.* But in a world where so many problems can be laid – either directly or indirectly

* This may be one of the most important reasons why the Theory has not yet fallen from grace. See *The Structure of Scientific Revolutions* by Thomas Kuhn (1962).

– at the feet of economics, to persist with policies based on a belief that is proven to be false is at a minimum peculiar, and at worst folly.

Real human beings have a thousand and one things to be thinking about and getting on with, and they simply don't have the time, energy, capacity or inclination to gather all the information necessary to make truly informed decisions.[9]

For big-ticket items, to be sure, the typical consumer spends more time investigating a product than they do for everyday or low-value items. But even in these cases there are limits. There is always a point where one says: enough – I have enough information in order to make this particular decision.

Now, if this decision was indeed rational, then the Theory might be OK. But the decision is almost never rational. Behavioural economics, for the last forty years or so (perhaps for even longer – it depends on who you believe), has been demonstrating with increasing potency that there is a simply staggering number of ways in which we humans can make decisions that are not rational.

Underpinning these numerous exceptions to the rule of rationality are the findings from cognitive science about how the human brain actually works. We have been evolving for millions of years in a universe in which there is a simply stupendous amount of information, only a very small fraction of which is actually useful. Useful, in evolutionary terms, means 'important for the purpose of finding food' or 'important for the purpose of finding a mate' or 'important for the purpose of avoiding being eaten'. It would be highly impractical to treat all information as having equal value – impractical not only in terms of the time it might take to run through a fully rational set of possibilities while a large-toothed predator sails through the air towards you, but impractical too in terms of the amount of blood-borne sugar required by the brain to run all the calculations. Instead we've evolved an entire skull-full of tricks to help us out.

These tricks – 'short cuts' in the vernacular, 'heuristics' in the technical jargon – include the defaults mentioned in the previous chapter; but there are many others. We are inordinately prone simply to copy what other people are doing rather than figuring it out for ourselves; we stop thinking about things as soon as we can and rely on habit instead; we make different decisions depending on how we've been primed (you can make people drive more safely just by showing them a picture of a baby[10]); we even, when confronted by identical circumstances, make different decisions on different days.

Rational? Consistent? It would seem not. And this sheds some interesting light on economics and all those people in the Treasury and the banks and the mega-corporations. You might suppose that evidence of a manifest flaw in one of your key underpinning shibboleths would give you cause to have something of a rethink; or, at least, to be a little more circumspect with your prognostications on the world. (Such was the hope of many, for example, in the aftermath of those awkward events in 2008.) Such a supposition would, however, be to misunderstand the degree of disassociation with which economists already operate.

For example, the Theory relies, as I've said, on the idea of the 'informed consumer'. This implies, obviously, that information that might be of relevance to the consumer should be made available to the consumer. That is why, as we saw earlier, we have to dodge all that information about the ingredients and the nutritional significance of our food every time we go to the supermarket. (Incidentally, don't worry if you really do never look at any of that stuff – hardly anybody else does; and if you think you *do* look at it, think again – researchers strapped eye-tracking machines to ordinary members of the public and were able to show that even people who claimed point-blank to have read the ingredients and the environmental credentials and the 'country of origin' information had only, in fact, looked at price and brand.[11])

And yet, information that is patently relevant – the amount of tax you're paying – is very obviously not made obvious. It has been mandated by government that the number of kilojoules is displayed, but not how much tax you're paying. Which is by way of saying that at least some of the economists in the Treasury have, for some reason, managed on this occasion to suspend their belief in the Theory and chosen not to inform the consumer.

Stranger still is that these very taxes, even if they were made transparent at the point of purchase, represent a transgression of the very belief system to which the economists are supposed to subscribe. An 'efficient market' should, according to the Theory, have no 'distortions': that is to say, the price you are required to pay for your chosen item should be solely the price that emerges from the interaction of all those competing suppliers and all those informed consumers. If a government places a tax on something, this efficiency is interrupted, misshaped, distorted, and the outcome is not, in fact, the most efficient one.

Believers in the Theory, therefore, already live with some disturbing incongruities: taxes that should not exist do; information that should be available is hidden. It is easy to understand how such minds are able to live with the idea that a fundamental assumption is wrong.

Interesting light is also thrown onto a branch of human endeavour that has not merely known about these frailties, foibles and inconsistencies of human behaviour for many years but has been ruthlessly exploiting this knowledge for our entire lives. Invented, in its modern incarnation, by Edward Bernays (a nephew of

Sigmund Freud) and called by him 'the engineering of consent', we know it today as 'marketing'.*

From the perspective of the Theory's believers, marketing and advertising are merely the provision of information. As they compete with one another for our custom, businesses issue information about their products; and we, striving hard to be as informed as possible, make use of this information in making our choices between the products and services on offer.

From the perspective of everyone else – and certainly anyone who has ever seen any advertising for a car, or a chocolate ice cream, or a fizzy drink containing quite startling amounts of sugar – marketing is a mechanism for evoking powerful emotions, for creating associations between fantastical imagined lifestyles and humdrum consumer choices, for creating a version of the world in which only certain choices make any sense. Competitive it may be; mere information it most certainly is not.

The defence from any organisation that is ever accused of manipulating the public in this way is that it is not possible for any single business to exert so much influence. Competition between entities, runs the argument, ensures that bad behaviours cannot persist. An organization that is systematically misleading its (actual and potential) customers will be found out, and it will lose custom and will either go bust or will have to

---

* I am using 'marketing' to refer to a broad range of dark arts – public affairs, corporate affairs, public relations and so forth.

reform. The Darwinian process (it may not be expressed quite like this) ensures that Good Things survive and Bad Things die out.

Two huge things are wrong with this. The first is the obvious one: it relies on the 'informed consumer' myth.

Second – and this is where things start to get really unsettling – it denies the existence of a wider social system within which all these businesses and consumers are operating; indeed, which they actually *comprise*.

To be fair, spotting a system is not easy; and figuring out how any particular system works, and why, is more difficult still. Most difficult of all is trying to discern the characteristics of a system from the inside, when all the available evidence and all the tools of analysis are themselves internal to the system. But the basic gist of social systems – other than the fact that they are complex – is twofold: everything is connected to everything else; and, because of this, there's nothing that can be unambiguously defined as the start or cause of something else. Everything in the system is both the cause of other things and the effect of other things.

Which means that, yes, it's true, any individual business cannot really be held responsible for marketing unhealthy products. It also means there really isn't anyone in particular to blame. That doesn't mean, however, that nothing can be done. There's something about the system as a whole – or, at a minimum, a big patch of the system – that somehow means that big businesses the world over consistently and continuously promote products that make us fat, that despoil the planet and that reinforce injustice and inequality. And there's something about the system that somehow also means that we consistently and continuously buy these things. We're as much to blame as they are.

Chapter 4

Whose choices are they?

Do not read beauty magazines, they will only make you feel ugly.

— *Mary Schmich*

We are, it is said, free to choose. Freedom and choice – what more could you want? There may be downsides to how modern liberal democratic economies work – climate change, systematic injustice, widespread mental illness and so forth – but the experience of feeling free, and being able to make our own choices as a result of that freedom, is enormously powerful.

If we cast our eye backward, the restraints and restrictions of the past appear profoundly uncomfortable. This is not to speak merely of consumer choice but to do so in a broader social and political sense. One need look back no further than the early 1970s, when VAT arrived in the UK, to get an intimation of how much has changed. Great swathes of the economy were still owned and controlled by the government; many prices and wages were controlled by the government too. Income taxes were high and so was inflation. The economy was being managed using the Keynesian techniques that had proven so effective in the immediate aftermath of World War II. Perhaps the overarching sense of the times was the 'collective': the social solidarity that put the Labour Party in power in 1945, that gave pre-eminence to 'us' rather than 'me', characterized the whole of the socio-economic system.

And this was reflected in the choices available to consumers, too. The blunt example of British Leyland illustrates the situation perfectly: here were cars that were built and designed not to meet the needs of the people that bought them but, rather, to meet the needs of the workers in the factories that built them, to meet the needs of the unions that represented those workers, and to meet the needs of the governments that owned the factories. So the cars were unreliable and poorly made and bad to drive? It mattered not.

It couldn't last, of course. Through the ever-more-enticing television screens came daily images of a land (in colour!) where people who looked just like us seemed to have a limitless supply of large and beautiful cars, of huge fridges stocked with unimaginably appetizing foods, of homes full of shiny and exotic furnishings and machinery. The American consumerist dream, seemingly inextricably linked with notions of personal freedom, tumbled relentlessly into British (and European and Soviet) lives, and the genie of choice escaped the bottle, forever.

And who would want it any other way? I, for one, am very keen on my personal freedom. I very much enjoy being able to make my own mind up and choose accordingly. I simply hate the idea of being told what to do.

The trouble is I'm not as free as I imagine. When I went shopping last week, it certainly felt, as I wandered the aisles, that there were many choices open to me. (I even enjoyed the feeling that there were other shops I could have chosen to visit for my groceries.) I stress the word 'felt', because there are three things I know to be true about these choices.

First, I am a frail human being with a brain that functions in a very particular way. I was riddled with defaults and biases as I wandered around the supermarket, my mind seething with a thousand and one preoccupations, my entire being a smoking cauldron of semi-conscious heuristics. I probably saw only a tiny fraction of the information presented to me: any recall I have about the experience will be in error; and the only reason I have any idea at all about how much I spent is because I made a special effort to keep the receipt.

Second, every single item in the shop is being presented to me as a choice only because someone somewhere thinks they can make a profit by selling it to me. In fact, I can be more specific still: those items upon which the profit margin is greatest – which just happen to be the items that have been most heavily processed[12] – are promoted to me more stridently than other items. (When was the last time you saw an end-of-aisle promotion for flour?) It is not so much that I am free to choose; it is, rather, that I am free to choose from within a broad but very strictly delimited set of options.

Third, my experience of choice has a direct relationship with my income. When I was poor, certain shops were simply off limits, and for any given item for which I may have been searching, certain brands were off limits too. Now that I am on a higher income, my choices have expanded. Now the obscure salads in M&S cross my choice horizon. Should my income ever go higher, I may choose to choose new choices.

In short, I may have felt as though I was free to choose in the supermarket but in reality I was extraordinarily constrained – by my brain, by the options made available by the capitalist system and by my income.

And millions of other people were similarly constrained.

If we wanted to overcome these constraints – if we wanted our freedom to be a little more real and a little less merely apparent – we'd have to tackle at least one of those three factors. To start with, it seems reasonable to suppose that there's not much we can do about how our brains work, not for the moment anyhow.

Tackling things at the level of income doesn't look promising, either. There is, to be sure, an ugly and shaming degree of inequality in modern Britain,[13] and one of

the most unjust features of such inequality is the extent
to which the choices available to the poor are so narrow
in comparison with those available to the wealthy. But
even a reduced disparity between the top and bottom
of the income spectrum would leave us with the same
pattern of constraint: the wealthy would still have more
choice(s) than the poor.

Which leaves us – for the moment at least – with
capitalism.

The increases in material well-being, in health and in
our ability to communicate and learn that have been delivered by the modern capitalist system are wonderful
and extraordinary. And there seems little doubt that the
Darwinian processes of competition and adaptation that
lie at the heart of the capitalist system have been instru-
mental in delivering these wonders.

Along with the wonders, however, there are worries.
In the case of my retail experience, and to use a jargon
term for a moment, there is a profound *asymmetry* in the
way choices are created and presented to us. Because
only some choices serve the interests of capitalism – that
is, only some choices are associated with profit, which is
the return (the reward, the prize) that capital requires –
many other possible choices are not presented, are not
available.

If the worst of this was merely a loss of freedom, then
perhaps it might not be worth worrying about. The issue
is that there is a direct connection between the nature

of the choices presented to us, on the one hand, and a whole host of big problems, on the other.

One of the most severe of these problems – in the UK and across the developed world – is obesity. There are many factors implicated in the obesity crisis: for example, scientists have identified the role played by genes[14] and the role played by the bacteria in our guts[15]. But there is no avoiding the fact that we, as a society, eat more calories than we need; and we eat too many of the fatty, sugary foods that make us fat. Why do we do this? At one level it's because we evolved to like these things in circumstances when they were rare. These days it's because far too many of the things presented to us to choose from have too much fat and sugar in them. And why is that? Because capitalist enterprises make more money from selling us things with fat and sugar in them than they otherwise would.

The economists have a word for problems like obesity: they call them 'externalities'. In doing what they do, capitalist enterprises have to pay all sorts of costs: the wages of the people they employ, the rent for the buildings they need, the diesel for the trucks they use to deliver all their products, and so forth. (Their simple mission, in the end, is to try to make sure that the total amount of money they receive from selling us things is greater than all these costs.) However, some of the costs that arise from their activities do not so easily fall within the perimeter of each individual enterprise; they are 'external' and hence are referred to as externalities.

Pollution is an externality: the poor air quality that is caused by all the diesel lorries imposes a cost on us, on society, and on the poor and the weak in particular.[16] It costs lives and millions, possibly billions, of pounds; but this is not paid for by the individual businesses, or even the industries that they comprise. It is paid for by society as a whole.

Climate change has been referred to as 'the mother of all externalities'.[17] Inequalities in income and wealth are externalities. A good deal of the stresses and strains that culminate in poor mental health are externalities. These are all costs that arise from capitalism but which are not paid by the businesses that cause them. It's true, of course, that these businesses only exist because modern consumers like you, me and millions of other people are buying the things that they produce, so in the end it's us that causes all these problems.* But – and this is why it really matters – we are not as free as we imagine. We only have certain choices presented to us, choices that cause these externalities. These choices are, in turn, presented and explained to us by the labyrinthine machinery of marketing, so much so that we are almost unable to even see it anymore.

---

* Strictly speaking it's the system as a whole that causes the problems – so the trick is to find the key 'leverage points' in the system where action has the potential to bring system-wide changes.

Two examples illustrate and hopefully explain some of this – one at either end of the spectrum.

Let's start with 'luxury brands'. Contemplate the two words that make up this phrase for a moment: 'luxury' and 'brand'. 'Brand' is a sign, a symbol, an indicator of something. It indicates, to the consumer, that a particular product (or service) is being made available by a particular provider. Since it is a symbol rather than a thing, a 'brand' is a message – or, more accurately, it is many messages. A brand conveys information, through its history, its associations, through the story of which it is a part. A brand, as part of a story, or a narrative, is therefore a thing about which a story is told, or made. The story you have in your head about Brand X (pick one you love, or hate, or notice within a few metres of wherever you now are) is just that: a story. And marketing has been the process by which you have been told that story, the whole of your life.

(Just as a brief thought experiment, ask yourself: do I even know the actual characteristics of the products that carry that brand? Do I know what it is made of, or how long it lasts, or where it was made? Yet you – we – are able to recall the story of the brand without any hesitation.)

From the point of view of mainstream (or orthodox) economics – the economics of the Theory – the key feature here is that word 'information'. Since the brand conveys information to consumers, it can be explained by the Theory as merely the way in which the brand owner helps to produce the 'informed consumer'. (It is important to remember that a brand is not the same as a company or business; a small number of companies each own many brands, so there are far fewer businesses than you might suppose on seeing the huge number of brands that fill the shelves.)

To the behavioural scientist, on the other hand, 'brand' is a short cut, a heuristic, a device that can be used by the consumer to avoid having to think. I buy, through habit, the same brand as I did last week, even if I am buying a different product. 'Brand loyalty' is the means by which I transfer the story from one item to another.

Stories are funny things. They exist in our heads. (They are members of the same family as myths.[18]) It has been suggested that the person that you think you are, your very identity, consists of the stories you tell yourself about who you are; you are a 'centre of narrative gravity'.[19] It has also been suggested that a culture or society can be defined and explained by means of the stories it tells about itself: the way in which you belong to a group, any group, is the process of having a story in common with other members of that group.[20]

So that sense of connection you fleetingly feel when you see someone reading the same newspaper, or wearing the same brand of shirt, or carrying the same branded bag – and this applies irrespective of the status of the paper, shirt or bag – is a moment of belonging, of having, of sharing the same story.

Marketing knows this. This is why car adverts no longer say anything about the car. Instead, they tell a story of how this particular car will enable you to express your idiosyncratic urban taste, or how you will be able to imagine the open winding road every time you sit in a traffic jam. Invented in the 1920s by Bernays, refined and commercialized on Madison Avenue in the 1960s, and now suffused through every pore of our consumerized culture, marketing does not sell products, it invents stories about 'lifestyles', stories that you carry around inside you until you think they are your own – so much so that when you are subjected to a promotion aimed at your 'target demographic', the product genuinely seems to fit exactly into your lifestyle choice. Oh, the irony: you express your individuality by buying a thing that's owned by millions of other people.

After a while, it has to be said, this process may become a little stale. That sense of individuality, of personal freedom, of identity that you got by expressing yourself through consumer choice starts to wear a little thin when you notice just how many other people seem to be carrying the same bag. (You want to belong to a group of people that 'feel' like you; perhaps they don't seem that way any more.) You want to differentiate yourself. You want ... a 'luxury brand'.

Luxury – what a fine word. What a fine idea! You've worked hard, you deserve a little special something; you deserve a luxury. And think of the stories! Luxury: fine silks and cushions; wine served from elegant decanters; an attentive factotum identifying your every wish just seconds before you even realised yourself that you needed – *needed* – a chocolate flavoured with genuine Madagascan vanilla. How else to signal to yourself and everybody else that you are acquainted with luxury than by buying a particular brand of watch, or a particular handbag?

We are a long way from meeting basic needs here. It is more than a century since Thorsten Veblen coined the phrase 'conspicuous consumption';[21] and there have been a few economists since then who have explored the way in which we humans seek to signal our status by the acquisition and display of what are called 'positional goods'.[22] But the general hope a hundred years or so ago – and it was a hope shared by Keynes[23] – was that we'd have gotten over all this by now. We'd have realized, they thought, that all this superficial shiny stuff signalled virtually nothing, merely that the person making the display had more money than sense. They hoped that, by now, we'd have realised that human virtue lies not in the choice of a watch or a chocolate or a bag, but in how we care for those we love, how we contribute to the improvement of life for those around us, how diligently we tackle the challenge of becoming wise. (See box 1.)

Box 1

Interestingly, when asked in a survey about such matters, the general public do acknowledge that money isn't everything.

Asked to what extent they agreed or disagreed with a series of statements, a representative sample of the population answered as follows.

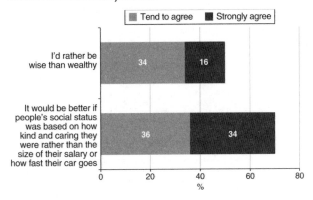

Questions were devised by the author; the survey was commissioned by Brook Lyndhurst and administered by GfK, online, with a representative sample of the UK adult population (n = 1,016) in autumn 2013.

What these economists failed to appreciate, however, was just how little reward capital accumulates from such activities, and how adept capital has been at inventing new ways to secure its rewards. In pursuit of those rewards, capital creates its very own '-ism' in the form of a self-sustaining spiral. For capital to accumulate more capital, it must make a surplus; for there to be a surplus – profit – there must be people spending money; for people to be spending money, they must have enough money to spend, and enough things to spend it on; and if they spend enough money on the right things, this enables enough jobs to be created paying enough money for them to carry on spending. Break any of the links, and the whole thing could come tumbling down.

So what to do when millions of people clearly have pretty much everything they need? It's time to start manufacturing wants, to 'engineer consent'. The product you bought last year – out of date! The shame! People will notice as you walk down the street, and you will feel like an outcast. And that shirt you bought – the wrong brand! Pariah!

'Luxury brands' are just the latest phase in the process by which you – we, I – are persuaded that we need to earn money so that we can spend money so that we can live the impossible story we unavoidably have in our head. We are not as free as we imagine. Only some choices are consistent with the perpetuation of capital and its -ism. Those are the choices we are offered and the stories we are told (sold).

Consider, by way of a second example and a contrast, the taking of a walk. Walking is an extraordinary and wonderful thing. It is blissfully simple – no special training is required. It is also marvellously equitable: it may seem that only a certain type or class of person 'goes for a walk' but, in fact, virtually all human beings can do it. You cannot walk better or worse by having loads of money or none.

Walking is good for the body, in both the short term and the long term. If everybody walked for just fifteen minutes a day, the rate of coronary heart disease – and all the pain and expense and distress that goes with it – would plummet.[24] (So, too, would our need for heart surgeons and, more especially, all those drugs we take to keep our tickers ticking.)

Walking is good for the mind, and individual well-being in the round.[25] Walking is good for our sense of collective well-being, too, for our communities: places where people walk rather than drive are friendlier and more convivial; they have more 'social capital'.[26]

And walking is good for the environment. When you walk, you emit no noxious fumes that might cause poor air quality; you use no valuable and irreplaceable resources; and you do not contribute to climate change.

So here we have a human activity which is unremittingly good – for you, your friends and family, all the people around you and the entire planet – that virtually everyone can do and which, astonishingly, is *completely free*.

And there's the rub. Consider how often this choice is promoted to you. You may, perhaps, have encountered a well-meaning initiative hidden somewhere on the NHS website.[27] But it is a flailing wave in an absolute ocean of inducements to drive, to fly, to catch a train, to drive

Box 2

People tend not to admit in surveys to behaviours of which they are ashamed, or about which they feel uncomfortable.

It is all the more remarkable, then, that so many people were ready to admit that they often eat more than they intended; that they so often buy things they didn't really want; and that they are so easily taken in by novelty.

Asked to what extent they agreed or disagreed with a series of statements, a representative sample of the population answered as follows.

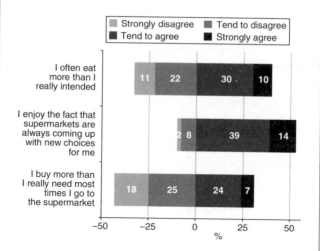

Questions were devised by the author; the survey was commissioned by Brook Lyndhurst and administered by GfK, online, with a representative sample of the UK adult population (*n* = 1,016) in autumn 2013.

some more. And why? Because it is almost impossible for anyone to make money – to make a profit – from people walking. Capital does not like it when you go for a walk, because it receives no reward. There is no return to capital. It has no interest in 'marketing' the idea of you going for a walk. It likes a story in which you imagine a wide curving road, leading to a deserted airport where you will have a luxury experience en route to a golden beach, perhaps even a yacht, where beautiful thin people in swimwear share cocktails and compare watches.

How odd it is. No matter how often we sit in traffic jams, or navigate crowded and uncomfortable airports, or find ourselves herded like cattle from one touristic experience to the next, these stories – these myths – persist in our heads. No matter how well we know that it is simply ridiculous to spend that much money on a single Belgian chocolate, no matter how well we understand that continuing to buy all this rubbish food will make us fat, still we wander into the supermarket and buy what they sell us. (See box 2.)

Is this really what we want?

Chapter 5

The stories we live by

> Imagining possibilities for ourselves involves telling stories about what we think we are like, what we think we want, and what we think we are capable of.
>
> — *Adam Phillips*

The economists do not believe that you know what you want. No, that's not quite right. They believe, rather, that what you want doesn't matter unless and until you actually make a choice. A transaction is where it becomes real for them. And there's a certain comfort in that: a choice expressed is a choice that's visible, that can be counted and measured. All those millions of people, free to choose, expressing what they want in a manner that can be measured: how reassuring.

As we have seen, however, the only choices that can be measured in this way are the choices made from the options that are available, and only certain kinds of options are presented. The economists live in a closed loop, in which proof of their rightness comes from the fact that they only deal with choices that exist within their frame of reference. Other choices, or possible choices, don't count, so they're not counted.

But, as the example of walking illustrates, there are other choices. And there are also ways of finding out what people want without waiting for them to buy something. You can ask them, for instance.

If you do actually ask people what they want – through a survey, for example – it turns out that people everywhere want the same relatively short list of things. They want health; and they want time with friends and family. They also – to cover the rest of the top five – want a nice house, a nice job and a nice environment.[28]

One has to be very careful with such lists, of course. There are many ways in which to ask questions in a survey, and many ways in which to elicit from a survey the answer that you're looking for. If you show a list of ten things and ask 'Which of these is most important to you?' that's different from if you show the same list and ask someone to rank them or to pick their top three.

The answers will be different, too, if you show a different list of ten things; and different again depending on whether you ask 'most important to you' as opposed to 'most important to you and your family', or just 'most important'; and different again if you ask 'most important in influencing your vote' or 'most important in choosing a holiday destination'.

To make matters still worse, there is invariably a gap – sometimes quite a big gap – between what people *say* is important to them and how they actually behave. A majority of people, for example, report to the nice people conducting surveys that they think the environment is important; but remarkably few people live environmentally friendly lives. Most people say they want the chickens to live happy lives before they become meat; that they want workers in other countries to be paid decent wages; and that they prefer to buy fruit and vegetables that have been grown 'locally'.[29] Needless to say, these same 'most people' – despite considerable effort on the part of well-meaning charities and government officials to come up with easy-to-understand labels[30] – carry on regardless, buying cheap chicken, unfair-trade coffee and air-freighted vegetables. (See box 3.)

Some of this gap occurs for the reasons we've already looked at: our little human brains are ceaselessly defaulting to our well-worn habits, so we too easily 'choose' the same brand we did last week; and marketing's surround-sound always points us to the brightly coloured offers and bargains (which are, just as they always are, the 'choices' that capital is interested in). (Do you think that capital receives more or less reward from locally grown vegetables than it does from air-freighted versions?)

But another part of the gap between what we say and what we do comes from the very different circumstances in which the saying and the doing take place.

Box 3

The public is prepared to admit that there is a gap between what they say is important and what they actually buy when they go to the shops. Asked how often they buy the most environmentally friendly option, they responded in the following way.

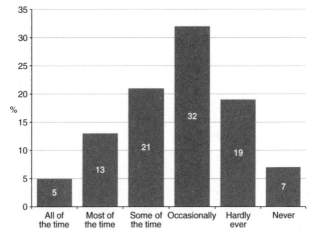

Questions were devised by the author; the survey was commissioned by Brook Lyndhurst and administered by GfK, online, with a representative sample of the UK adult population (*n* = 1,016) in autumn 2013.

The 'doing' always take place in a shop or a showroom or (increasingly) on-line, and the doing is the expression of *consumer* choice. We are, in such circumstances, functioning in a particular mode, playing a very particular role – listening to and being a part of a very particular story. We are Consumer, free to choose, and we behave accordingly.

When we are asked a question by a nice researcher we are very frequently in our homes, on our sofa, on the telephone; or perhaps even on our sofa talking to them face to face. (I know this not least because I have been that nice researcher on the phone or in your living room.) Increasingly, such surveys are conducted on-line, so people (in the jargon, 'respondents') may at first sight appear to be doing something very similar to shopping. In fact, as your own experience will attest, there are very different ways of being in front of a computer screen: you are in a very different mode when, say, searching on-line for a holiday compared with playing *Warcraft*; and different again if looking at titillating photos compared with trying to find out how to repair the toaster.

Irrespective of the mode used to ask you the questions, you respond as your better self – as the good citizen you want yourself to be. No one wants to think of themselves as a bad person; few people are either confident or comfortable enough to tell the nice researcher (a fellow human being, after all) that they behave terribly, or that they consider something they 'know' to be important to be a total waste of time. Imagine: 'Frankly, I think polar bears are totally overrated and I can't wait for them to become extinct.' There may be a freakish few willing to say this out loud, but the power of the 'injunctive norm' is great and the majority of us, even if we think it, would not say it. (And here is why the differences in the mode of questioning are so relevant:

the online world, so often anonymized, eliminates the power of the injunctive norm, freeing us to troll, vent splenetically and lie in new ways to pollsters.)

What is interesting here is how we all 'know' what the 'right' answer is; that is, what is the means by which we absorb the injunctive norm? Let's try something like the following: we are powerfully driven by our evolutionary urge to be social, to 'belong', to be part of a group. We touched earlier on how we might express that belonging by the acquisition of the right brands. Belonging is the sharing of the same story as others of the same group or tribe. The brand is a sign of a shared story. Even the simplest story operates on many levels and, centres of narrative gravity that we are, we learn extraordinarily early on in our lives how to tell whether something is or is not consistent with the story we are being told. A story contains within itself its own rules, invariably implicitly, and our brains figure out the rules virtually subconsciously.[31]

The process of becoming a member of modern society – of learning how to belong to society – means absorbing an interlocking set of stories. These stories are internally consistent, and the rules tell us how to behave: that is, they tell us how to behave in such a way as to remain a member of the group. This belonging is, for most people and most of the time, both the easiest and the safest thing to do. (All of this, needless to say, is the outcome of millions of years of thoroughly impressive evolutionary effort.) These rules are the injunctive norms. They are component parts of the 'deep frames'[32] upon which our stories are built.

In the story you tell yourself of the good person that you are, you are Citizen, a member of society. In this story, you always drive sensibly, you never drink too much and you help old ladies across the street. You recycle as much as you can, never leave the tap running when you brush your teeth and always switch the light off when you leave the room.

This is very different from how things are when you are Consumer. As Consumer, you are in a hurry, you are thinking about what your partner and/or children will or will not eat, you are worrying about how long you have before the bus leaves or the ticket expires, you cannot remember whether there's enough milk in the fridge and, since you don't really know what you might eat on Friday, you are very tempted by that offer of some bits of chicken and vegetables with the sauce already added that you'll only need to throw in the oven.[33] As your hand deposits two packets into the trolley (you don't really need two, but that's the only way to get the special offer) you have no idea at all and don't really care where the chicken or the vegetables came from, or whether they or anyone involved in their production lived a happy life.

As Citizen, listening to the nice researcher's questions, the story comes effortlessly. Of course these things matter to you.

It's not that you or the millions of other people are lying. As Citizen, you know that all those fatty foods are bad for you. You know – everyone knows – that it really isn't a good idea to drink all those sugar-in-suspension fizzy drinks, to eat so much salt and red meat and dough-nuts. As Consumer, they all seem so tempting. As fragile animal, still driven by all those evolutionary millennia in your bewildered and bewildering brain, it's so easy to eat them: just one more chocolate…

Not everyone does this all the time, of course; and virtually all of us have had the experience of 'resisting temptation'. To a greater or lesser extent, we assert 'self-control'[34] in the face of the onslaught. Marketing – armed to the teeth with weapons-grade tools of ma-nipulation and swaggering with the confidence borne of approaching a century's experience under its belt – bom-bards us with emotion-laden stories intended to ensure we choose only from the choices that serve the interests of capital and its -ism; we, by and large, succumb, and we become fatter and fatter. Sometimes, on an idle Tuesday, we have had enough; and we pledge to stop smoking, drinking and eating ready meals. We pledge to stop giv-ing in to our children's demands for the latest ridiculous drink they've seen advertised; we pledge to give them apples instead of chocolates; we pledge to cook them a proper meal rather than throw some sauce-smothered, additive-riddled, fat-laden ready meal in the microwave. (See box 4.)

Box 4

Again, the survey results reveal not only a gap between what people say they want and what they say they do, but also an awareness of the gap.

Asked to what extent they agreed or disagreed with a series of statements, a representative sample of the population answered as follows.

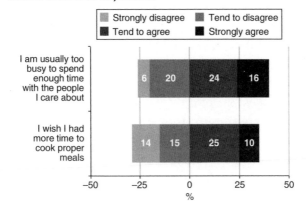

Questions were devised by the author; the survey was commissioned by Brook Lyndhurst and administered by GfK, online, with a representative sample of the UK adult population (n = 1,016) in autumn 2013.

And, wonderfully, sometimes we succeed. How?

The name for what we do is a 'commitment device'. Coined by the marvellous Thomas Schelling,[35] the phrase refers to a mechanism by which the today-you imposes a constraint on the tomorrow-you. Setting your alarm for the morning is a commitment device: today-you knows that, unless something stops you, tomorrow-you will sleep blissfully until lunchtime. By setting the alarm, today-you imposes an obligation to wake at a particular time on tomorrow-you.

Taking a shopping list to the supermarket is a commitment device. (My first economics teacher explained that going to the supermarket without a shopping list was tantamount to 'economic suicide'.) The you that sits calmly at the kitchen table to write a list of things you need is sending instructions, and thus restrictions, to the you that will be ambling up and down the aisles of enticement in an hour or two. Citizen-you is sending instructions to Consumer-you.

Limiting your options for spending too much by visiting your local stores rather than Oxford Street is a commitment device. Setting yourself a spending limit before you even leave the house is a commitment device. Writing on your hand the words 'Buy the low-fat version' is a commitment device. Cutting up your credit card so that you are simply unable to indulge in some retail therapy is a commitment device.

You can immediately see two things. Commitment devices come in differing strengths; and different behaviours require different devices. Head to the supermarket with a scrappy list and you are only lightly defended against the onslaught; you will still need considerable will-power to enforce the commitment. Head to the mall without a credit card, and it will be really quite difficult to spend much money.

Head to the supermarket without any plastic, on the other hand, and feeding yourself and your family would become difficult, which is rather the opposite of what one might be after. Similarly, heading to the mall with a list that says 'handbag, watch' is unlikely to protect you from all those luxury brands.

Schelling himself thought first about smoking – indeed, his own smoking – and initially extended his thinking to other compulsive behaviours that we humans seem so keen on. Virtually everyone has some sort of ongoing battle, with smoking or chocolate or gambling or alcohol or picking their nails or ... (insert your own personal demon here, should it not already have been listed). And virtually everyone will have, on one or (more probably) many occasions, invented some sort of commitment device in an attempt to restrict or abandon their ugly behaviour. The you of yesterday tried really hard to come up with a cunning plan, but the you of today still found a way to have a crafty fag or slip in a bonus doughnut.

As we also know, however, sometimes these commitment devices actually work. And it turns out there are some relatively straightforward features that distinguish effective devices from ineffective devices. They need to be easy to use, for example; and they need to have their effect at the right time. By some margin the most important feature that distinguishes the effective from the ineffective, however, is the extent to which it is public rather than private. In general, a commitment device that is devised by a group and then operates in a public fashion will be more effective than a device devised by an individual and applied in isolation.

If we think about food again, for a moment, simply consider the difference between you personally deciding to reduce the number of ready meals you eat each week and a decision by your entire household to eat fewer ready meals. You can immediately *feel* that not only would you individually find it harder to continue eating so many ready meals if no one else in the household was doing so, but the whole household would find it easier to stop eating such rubbish if they had all agreed together than if each of them had decided separately.

You can also quickly see a link to the injunctive norms we were discussing earlier. Norms, remember, are the rules that govern membership of the group. Commitment devices constitute new rules.

Schelling took this line of thinking the whole way. He re-presented 'law' as commitment devices. A legal statute – let's say something like 'it is illegal to drive a car whilst under the influence of alcohol' – is the people of yesterday imposing a restriction on the people of today (us). Social institutions, too, have this character: the way a museum presents a particular cultural view of the world, the way a parliament presents a particular way of conducting debate, the way money presents a particular way of conducting exchange – all are inventions of past peoples, and act to shape and constrain the way the peoples of tomorrow see, think and behave.

And in the same way that your shopping list or diced credit card may or may not work – may or may not be appropriate – so too with human laws and institutions. Sometimes the people of yesteryear got it wrong and we need to amend or replace their commitment devices; the progressive repeal in recent years of the various laws against homosexuality would be a good example.

Thinking about it from this slightly bigger and longer-term perspective gets us towards the idea of a 'commitment strategy'. Stopping an entire country smoking, for example, is the kind of thing that you can't really do in one go. You are probably going to need a whole host of mechanisms or 'interventions' or commitment devices. A commitment strategy is a plan for such a situation, where a range of commitment devices will be necessary and where it will be important to think about which devices get used to achieve which outcomes at which times.

Note, again, the importance of the group dynamic in all this. The commitment device known as 'banning smoking in public places' would have been impossible in the UK ten or twenty years earlier because smoking was still too prevalent: it was still sufficiently widespread to have the character of an injunctive norm. It was something that was a key part of the story of being a member of the group called 'society'. By 2007, when the ban actually came into effect, smoking rates had fallen to levels whereby a sufficiently large majority of people did not smoke, to the point where the injunctive norm had flipped. The story had changed.

Throwing all this together, this thing we call 'British society' looks like a tangle of inherited commitment devices, broadly devised and implemented in a public fashion, evolving slowly, and carried around in our heads as a more-or-less tangible story that contains the rules of how to behave. In general, and certainly if they're going to be successful, new rules – new commitment devices – are considered and devised by our better selves, with the specific intention of trying to restrict the weaker selves that we know we will at some point be tomorrow, or the day after.

Which gets us back to shopping. Millions of us believe, and routinely tell the nice researchers, that our health is our top priority. Yet we buy and eat a simply astonishing amount of food that makes us ill. We eat food that harms our hearts, clogs our arteries, gnaws away at several vital organs and makes us fat. The main reason we do this is not that we're stupid; it's not even that there is always a gap between what we say and what we do. It's because we are subjected to a sophisticated and unremitting assault from all sides: a surround-sound of interwoven stories that has been saturating our mammal minds for so long that we barely even notice it any more.

We inhabit an environment in which ever more aspects of our lives require us to fulfil the role of Consumer, a role in which we experience an intoxicating sense of choice, but in which only choices that serve the interests of capital are presented. The asymmetry is acute; and we have not yet put in place the strategies, devices or tools to redress the imbalance.

So what if, rather than each of us battling on our own to eat the right amount of fruit, avoid the fatty rubbish, cut back on the chocolate, stop drinking the fizzy drinks, and so on and so forth – what if instead we decided to do it together? What if, as Citizens today, we agreed on some commitment devices to control our Consumer selves tomorrow?

What might such commitment devices look like?

Chapter 6

How we make new commitments

I fought the law, and the law won
— *Sonny Curtis*

I f we follow Schelling's lead and think about the ways in which societies impose commitment devices upon their future selves, we find the same three types of 'policy instrument' I mentioned in chapter 2.

- *Regulatory*: we can pass laws to ban certain foods, or certain ingredients, or certain food-preparation practices, for example.
- *Persuasion*: we can try to encourage businesses to work together to change the amount of salt or sugar they put into their food; and we can try to encourage people to make different choices, with information campaigns and behaviour-change strategies and so on.

- *Fiscal*: we can use money, by increasing or decreasing the price of things, or fining or incentivizing people and businesses.

If we think about the way in which smoking has been tackled over the past forty or fifty years, we can see how it has comprised a commitment strategy using all three of these types of device. The price of cigarettes has been increased in fits and starts by Chancellors of the Exchequer imposing special taxes called 'duties'; there have been innumerable campaigns to highlight the negative health consequences of smoking, ranging from mass media advertising to the display of graphic images on cigarette packets to highly tailored behaviour-change campaigns aimed at particular (and stubborn) target groups; and, as we saw earlier, legislation has been used to ban smoking in public places.

In the case of smoking, the science supporting the assertion that it was bad for you built slowly, and was – let us not forget – resisted powerfully by the tobacco lobby.[36] It is worth noting, too, that although there is some variety in the ways it is possible to consume tobacco, it is a relatively well-defined and identifiable activity.

Food, by contrast, is a very different case. The scientific evidence in support of the assertion that, say, 'eating too much sugar is bad for you'[37] is as incontrovertible as similar assertions about tobacco, but the number of ways of ingesting too much sugar is enormous. The type and power and mix of commitment devices we might need will necessarily be different compared with tobacco.

Using legislative instruments to reduce sugar intake (to continue the example) would appear doomed from the start. There are too many variables, too many complications, too many obvious difficulties. We are not going to be able to ban our way to health.

Using the tools of persuasion would appear to be more appealing; and this is indeed where such efforts have focused so far. There has certainly been progress with salt,[38] for example: UK and European governments have worked with major food producers and suppliers (through what are called 'Voluntary Agreements') to progressively reduce the amount of salt in a wide range of foods. And on the consumer side, too, programmes such as 'Change for Life'[39] have demonstrated some success.

Voluntary Agreements – soft commitment devices in which a group of businesses and one or more government agencies work together towards mutually agreed goals – are nevertheless highly limited. They tend to work when the goals are sufficiently consistent with the general objectives of capital. Voluntary Agreements to reduce energy consumption or resource use, for example, which government pursues on environmental grounds, have the happy side effect of also helping to reduce the costs of production, so businesses are happy to play along. As soon as core interests are threatened – as soon as the big scary businesses start sucking their teeth and explaining how difficult it will be, their tooth-sucking the sign that capital and its -ism are not happy – then progress comes to an end. Progress on salt came to a halt as soon as one or two major corporations suggested that any further reductions might be noticed by consumers (that is, that their consumers might stop buying so many of whatever they were selling). Progress on reducing alcohol consumption and sugar has so far been risible for similar reasons.

Perhaps this would be acceptable if the problems we face were more modest in scale: but the health problems associated with the food we eat are huge and worsening; and the costs, both personal and social (and environmental!), are enormous. At the same time, the persuasive tools at our disposal are too weak, too soft and work too slowly. Voluntary Agreements and behaviour-change programmes are homemade pea shooters in the face of the weapons-grade onslaught of contemporary marketing.

Which brings us to the money. There have recently been suggestions that we have a 'fat tax'[40] or a 'sugar tax'[41] or a 'minimum unit price'[42] on alcohol. As we saw back in chapter 2, it is close to an iron rule that, if the price of something goes up, the amount we buy goes down. If each gram of fat in the burger or the ready meal had a tax on it, and there were some less fatty alternatives available, then it would be reasonable to expect sales of the former to go down and the latter to go up. Which would be good.

But not good enough. If we focus on fat, what about the sugar? If we focus on sugar, what happens to our consumption of fruit and vegetables? If we have a 'fat and sugar tax', what about additives, or any of the dozens of other things that might harm us if we swallow too much?

Then there's the challenge (frequently) raised by the manufacturers of certain sugar-in-suspension fizzy drinks that there is no such thing as an unhealthy item of food, only an unhealthy diet. What they mean by this is that the relationship between your health and your diet is precisely that: it's a relationship between your body (and mind) and the *entirety* of what you eat, not an individual item. Strictly speaking, this is true: if my healthy weekly intake of sugar is X, and this can of sugar-in-suspension supplies precisely that amount, then I am clearly not exceeding my healthy limit if I drink it. All I need to do is to make sure that I avoid sugar for the rest of the week and I'll be fine.

And of course the very word 'healthy' is problematic. If you are a petite and relatively inactive middle-aged female, the diet that would be healthy for you looks very different from the diet necessary to keep a hulking teenage male athlete in good shape. We might generalize for the purposes of providing Guideline Daily Amounts on the side of our breakfast cereals, but how on earth could we devise a commitment device that would be fair to the extraordinary diversity of different people, different foods and different diets?

This complexity has been the reason that so little progress has been made. With most of the externalities created by the food choices we are offered being either far in the future, or dispersed, or difficult to see, the pressure to grasp the nettle has not yet been strong enough.

But that nettle must surely be grasped at some point. The solution, just as surely, must be based on the acknowledgement that we need a serious commitment device for a serious problem. The solution that is both the simplest and the most serious is to change the relative prices of good and bad diets. Our commitment strategy should be to decrease the price of healthy food and increase the price of food that makes us unhealthy.

Remarkably, a mechanism for doing this already exists; and it is a mechanism that, as we saw earlier, is opaque, woefully out of date and badly in need of an overhaul. We should use the VAT system. We should impose VAT on bad foods – and apply negative VAT to healthy foods.

Chapter 7

Changing our minds

Enlightenment is man's emergence from his self-imposed immaturity.
Immaturity is the inability to use one's understanding without guidance from another.
Have courage to use your own understanding!
— *Immanuel Kant*

I spent much of the last chapter suggesting that 'we' should devise a commitment strategy to help us choose, and eat, healthier foods. By the end of the chapter I had suggested that there should be high(er) VAT on bad foods and negative VAT on healthy foods. Perhaps the most conspicuous difficulty with this proposition is that it is not 'we' that impose VAT, it is government.

At one time, perhaps, the relationship between the citizens of the UK and their government was sufficiently close for this not to be an issue. Once, perhaps, the story of our society and the stories each individual carried around in their head contained enough of the language and concepts of conviviality and collaboration, of community and cooperation, that our government really did feel like an extension of us. Perhaps this is how it felt immediately after World War II, when the manifestation of collective endeavour was so obvious, when the needs of our brothers and sisters were so apparent. Certainly the Welfare State, created by the Labour government elected in 1945, seems to have such sentiments embedded in its DNA. The Welfare State is a marvellous example of a commitment strategy; and 'we' built it through the agency of 'our' government.

In these early decades of the twenty-first century, however, it can no longer be claimed that a government could act in such a way. A full account of why this is so lies beyond the scope of this book, but the rise of individualism (itself interwoven with the rise of consumerism), the collapse in the trust that the general public has in its elected representatives[43] and the growing complexity of the challenges that government is expected to tackle[44] would all appear to be implicated. A government in the 1940s or 1950s – and perhaps the 1960s or even the 1970s – might have been able to make an argument that taxes needed to be increased in order to address some society-wide problem. A modern government seems to have no such room for manoeuvre. Indeed, the idea of increasing taxes for any reason whatsoever seems to be becoming politically untenable.

There are other problems with the idea of increasing the price of unhealthy foods. Some, perhaps many, will think it unfair. Why should the people that simply want to eat those things be penalized? It may be, for example, that it is mainly people on low incomes that buy these items, so it would be the poor that suffered most – something that would very definitely be unfair.

The priests and acolytes of the Theory won't be happy either: they believe that such taxes would be a distortion of the market, leading to inefficient outcomes for the economy as a whole.

The big scary companies that make all the unhealthy foods would definitely be unhappy. They will explain that they invest enormous sums of money in researching and developing new food products, and all they are trying to do is meet the fickle tastes of consumers. They will show how many of their products are unsuccessful; how many of their products are healthy; how hard they try to work with 'stakeholders'. They will commission research and publish reports and organize press releases and fund lobbying processes – in short, they will mimic their normal marketing strategies – in order to show that a tax reform of this kind would mean calamity. They will show how tax revenue would fall, how employment would fall, how consumers would be angry and distressed. They would devote simply astounding resources to terrify the living daylights out of the politicians whose job it would be to implement a change of this kind.

At no point would they admit that the only reason they are cross is because they might not make quite so much money and therefore might not be able to deliver unto capital the rewards it requires.

These are formidable challenges. Any solution is going to need to be able to address all of them. There are two reasons why I am convinced that such a solution is possible.

The first reason – as I hope the remaining chapters will persuade you – is that the solution I happen to be putting forward is based on assembling a set of mechanisms each of which has been implemented successfully somewhere or somewhen else. It may be that the solution I propose is not, in the end, the best solution; and even if it is, there may be another solution that for one reason or another is the one that is implemented. But the very fact that I can imagine one solution that can be put into practice means that there is at least one, and there may be more.

The second reason I'm convinced a solution is possible is because of what I've had the opportunity to witness over a working lifetime of research. Predominantly by luck rather than judgment I have spent time with the leaders of big businesses, with politicians and ministers, with food scientists and policy wonks. I've spent time with economists and statisticians, and with experts in health and diet. I've also spent time – lots of time – talking with ordinary members of the public: on the phone, in their living rooms and in focus groups.

One of the most striking common features of my discussions with all of these different groups of people is the difference between the assumptions that are made about them and what they are really like. All too often – and, given our limited brains, this sort of thing is understand-able – we have somewhat crude, occasionally unpleasant, stereotypical images in our heads. Food scientists have big brains and wear white coats. Politicians have big ex-pense accounts and bigger egos. Business folk are greedy people with leather chairs and sharp elbows.

Most of all, and worst of all, it is a widespread view that 'the general public' (that is, everyone else apart from whoever is speaking at the time and whoever they're speaking to) holds a set of simplistic beliefs about the world, is generally reactionary and cannot be relied upon to understand any argument that cannot be reduced to a sound bite.

In my experience, ordinary people have got plenty to deal with on a day-to-day basis and do not always have or make the time to ensure that they have a well-thought-through opinion on each and every subject. Even if they do have a well-thought-through opinion, it is in all likeli-hood an opinion formulated at some point in the past and is therefore quite possibly out of kilter with not only the actual facts in the world but possibly also the myriad other beliefs and opinions scattered throughout their mind. And, of course, since we are all ordinary people, this applies to you and me too.

As we saw earlier when discussing the insights from behavioural economics, the utterly normal solution to the problem of there being far too much information and nowhere near enough time is to develop short cuts, or heuristics, upon which we can rely to get by. Another way of describing the same process is that we rely on myths – fragments of stories that live within our bigger stories of belonging – to handle the stuff we find too demanding or complex or impenetrable. Most of our opinions are like this: relatively untested myth fragments, with a mix of evidence and guesswork to complete the story.

Whenever people are invited to spend some time actually reflecting on an issue, however, the situation changes. When the nice researcher asks a single blunt question, the respondent does not rely on only the injunctive norm that they know will evoke a favourable response from the interviewer; the respondent also relies on the story fragment or myth or heuristic that has been lodged in their brain since whenever it arrived. This adds to the dangers of surveys outlined earlier.

Given time to reflect upon and discuss their initial response, many people discover that they change their minds, particularly on complicated or sensitive issues. In the right environment – by which I principally mean a setting where people are not made to feel ashamed at admitting to changing their mind – this process can be powerful for both the individual and other people with whom they might be engaging. It has been my experience, particularly in focus groups and discussion groups, that people can, in general, progress from knee-jerk (often negative) reactions to sophisticated (sometimes positive) reactions, and can sometimes do so relatively quickly. (I have witnessed the same behaviour among business leaders, scientists and politicians.) The very process of being given the time to discuss an issue and being invited to do so is the thing that was absent from their day-to-day lives. (Where might they have such a discussion? With whom? It surely cannot be said, as the media so often seems to do, that a 'public discussion' has taken place when one extreme position or another is assumed, adopted and then shouted via a headline.)

This observation does not, thankfully, rely exclusively upon my experience. The terms 'deliberative research' and 'deliberative democracy' have been coined to describe it; and there is a significant body of strong academic work that shows just how far opinion can shift during the course of a deliberative process.[45] Done thoroughly and well, deliberative processes have two key features: firstly, they enable participants from all social backgrounds to participate fully and on a fair footing; and, secondly, they entail the gathering, presentation and testing of evidence – evidence that directly addresses the issues and questions raised during the discussion.

Which is all by way of saying that whilst transforming VAT from an antiquated money-raising tool into a twenty-first century commitment device might at first sight seem like the sort of thing that will be rejected out of hand by virtually everyone, maybe it just seems that way because we haven't given people the opportunity to think it through.

Chapter 8

The story so far

> The art of progress is to preserve order amid change,
> and to preserve change amid order.
> — *Alfred North Whitehead*

Let us summarize the argument so far.

Economic policy in the UK, and across most of the rest of the developed world, is based predominantly upon the belief that free and competitive markets always deliver the best possible outcomes. A key tenet of this theory is belief in the 'informed consumer', a version of 'rational economic (hu)man'.

The Theory proposes that, so long as consumers are provided with sufficient and accurate information, they will make the decisions necessary to ensure that the overall results – in terms of what things get made, what things cost, how many jobs there are and so on – are the most economically efficient possible.

Human minds have developed a range of systematic biases during the course of their evolution that help us to cope with the challenges of everyday life. Foremost among these are various mental short cuts, or heuristics. These heuristics are so deeply embedded and so widespread that consumers cannot, in reality, play the role expected of them by the Theory. The 'informed consumer' is a myth.

Humans rely on myths and stories all the time. We use them to understand the world around us, to tell ourselves who we are and to know the rules of the society to which we belong so that we can act as good citizens.

Our modern society is dominated as never before by sophisticated marketing. Marketing does not simply promote products that people might buy; it constructs entire narratives about lifestyles and aspiration. These narratives and stories – these myths – have been comprehensively internalized by citizens, to the point where the principal means for self-expression for large numbers of people is in their role as consumer.

The machinery of marketing emphasizes the importance of individual choice, connecting to a powerful human story of freedom and personal agency. However, despite the apparent abundance of choice, only certain options are made available by marketing. Those options are the products and services that deliver, or are expected to deliver, a return to capital.

The power and sophistication of modern marketing creates a dramatic asymmetry in the structure of choice. Choices that do not provide a return to capital are marginalized – both directly, by having fewer resources available to promote them, and indirectly, by being made to appear inconsistent with the dominant themes of the stories that shape social belonging.

The problems arising from this state of affairs are considerable. Economists call these problems – these harms – externalities. Climate change is perhaps the most dramatic: it is primarily the 'Western lifestyle' (in terms both of those that have one and those that want one) that drives the emissions that are propelling climate change; and central to the very notion of 'Western lifestyle' are the myths created and maintained by modern marketing. (Indeed, the very word 'lifestyle' is mythological, and was itself coined in the 1920s for marketing purposes.)

Extreme inequality is almost certainly exacerbated by this asymmetry – the preposterous 'luxury brands' and their ilk encourage us to run fast, and the fast to run faster, and the faster to run faster still, stretching the distribution of income and wealth ever wider. It is likely, too, that a goodly share of our ever-burgeoning psychological disorders are fuelled at least in part by the requirements of aspiration, as we desperately strive to live the stories that we have come to believe will enable us to belong and to be held in high esteem. And if that's true, then responsibility for the harm caused by our innumerable compensations – the drugs, the alcohol, the gambling – can also be placed at the same door.

And obesity, too. As I've said, there are other factors at play, to be sure: sedentary lifestyles, the kinds of bugs we have in our gut, a bit of genetics. But the allure of the cheap, sugary, easy, convenient fatty foods – the same foods that are most attractive to capital and its -ism – is too great; and there's even a dark twist, given that many of us eat these foods for comfort, as compensations for the stresses and strains placed upon us by the sundry other tentacles of the marketing beast.

It feels increasingly odd to say that we 'want' these things. We want a luxury brand, a new television, a lovely cake. But we do not want climate change. We do not want to be driven mad. We do not want to be obese.[46] The myths of marketing fulfil wants that are immediate; capital is not interested in things that are too far away (except insofar as it will be able to convert the future need to *overcome* these harms into profit-making opportunities, by selling us pills and surgery).

Given the opportunity to express what they want in settings that are not under the total control of modern marketing, people say that they want to be healthy and that they want to spend time with their friends and family. They may even want to go for a walk.

A useful distinction is between the expression of wants as a Citizen and as a Consumer. The former wants to be healthy and well; the latter eats the stuff promoted by the marketing myth, and gets fat.

The techniques used by individuals and entire societies to stick to the promises they make to themselves are called commitment devices. Promises made by the you (us) of today are imposed on the you (us) of tomorrow. The thoughtful Citizen of today *knows* that smoking is bad; and knows, too, that the person they will be tomorrow will struggle to resist the temptation to smoke. An effective commitment device – or, if there are multiple devices, a commitment strategy – is one that is precisely tailored to the temptation. A Citizen of today that wishes to eat well and not become obese needs to develop a commitment strategy to control the Consumer of tomorrow as he or she attempts to navigate the labyrinth created by modern marketing.

Collective commitment strategies take the form of laws and institutions. Their effectiveness depends on similar factors as apply to the individual: they need to be precisely tailored to the particular circumstance.

In the case of a collective process, societies have long relied on politics. (It is possible to construe 'politics' as the process by which a society reflects upon and refines its commitment strategies.) A society – that is to say, the individuals that comprise that society – needs to believe in a commitment device if it is to work.

Public confidence in an increasingly elite representative politics has now fallen to such an extent that it is hard to envisage certain kinds of commitment device being formulated through the traditional mechanisms. Publics simply do not trust their governments any more. The idea of deliberative democracy, and of deliberative processes more generally, has emerged to fill this developing void.

Finally, elementary economics teaches us that, by and large, the amount we buy of something is linked directly to its price. If something becomes more expensive, we tend to buy less; if it becomes cheaper, we tend to buy more.

Which leads us to the following proposition.

To tackle the obesity crisis, we need a collective commitment strategy. This strategy needs to rebalance the asymmetry created by modern marketing. The most powerful tool by which we might influence our choices is price. Merely to increase the price of some foods would be inadequate and unfair. The most powerful commitment device would be to *reduce* the price of healthy foods and to *increase* the price of unhealthy foods.

A mechanism for affecting the price of food already exists – it is called value added tax. This tax is already woefully out of date and in need of a profound overhaul.

Taxes are generally unpopular; so too are governments. It is hard to imagine that a modern government, of any hue, could begin increasing taxes on food. A broad, inclusive and transparent deliberative process, on the other hand, may offer a solution. Taxes may be unpopular, but Citizens generally acknowledge that they are necessary. If taxes were to transparently play the role of a commitment device – a device by which the Citizens of today rescue the Consumers of tomorrow – it is very possible that a way forward could be found.

Chapter 9

The start of a new story

Two types of choices seem to me to have been crucial in tipping the outcomes [of the various societies' histories] towards success or failure: long-term planning and willingness to reconsider core values.

— *Jared Diamond*

The devil of the commitment strategy proposed in the preceding chapter is very much in the detail. So let's go through the detail step by step.

Step 1 of 4

The crucial first step will be to decide which foods are healthy and which are unhealthy.

As I mentioned earlier, there is a view that there is no such thing as an 'unhealthy' food item, only an unhealthy diet. A bottle of sugar-suspended-in-fizzy-water, so long as you manage the rest of your weekly intake, is clearly not lethal. So it is possible to claim that virtually any individual food item is not, in and of itself, 'unhealthy'. Such arguments are, of course, made most routinely by the enterprises that manufacture such items and who, as we know, are interested in serving capital.

These enterprises have nevertheless acceded (slowly, of course) to the idea that some sort of nutritional information should be made available on their products so that the 'informed consumer' can make sensible dietary choices. (This is why the information about how much sugar is actually suspended in the fizzy liquid is made so obvious. Not.) These nutritional facts and figures are established using scientific methods – and the evidence from science is, of course, information *par excellence*.

It is an easy and natural assumption that decisions about 'healthy' or 'unhealthy' should be based on the science; indeed, that they should be based *exclusively* on the science. And if we were conducting a scientific experiment, then that would be fine. But that's not what we're doing here. We are constructing a commitment device. A commitment device is not a scientific experiment or a scientific instrument – it is a human construct, made from belief and judgment and imagination. More formally, it is *vernacular*. If we decide, as part of our commitment strategy, to put food A in the good category and food B in the bad category, that's really our lookout. It would be fairly straightforward: a group of people are somehow nominated or selected to choose on our collective behalf, they participate in a deliberative exercise to choose what goes where, and hey presto!

This approach doesn't seem entirely convincing. Completely excluding the reality of scientific information is simply foolhardy. (It is precisely the obverse of the current foolhardiness, in which the reality of how people really are is excluded.) Some sort of hybrid is required.

And this, remarkably enough, is exactly how deliberative processes actually work. A group of citizens is selected or invited to participate, just as when conducting a survey, and they are, typically, invited firstly to air their opinions and beliefs (about the matter at hand) in a fairly unstructured fashion. The moderators – the people organizing the process – take a look at everything that's been said, organize it into bundles of questions, and then go looking for people that might be able to address those questions. Typically, again, these people are 'experts' of some sort. The citizens are then reconvened and they have the opportunity to quiz the experts directly. Similarly, the experts have the opportunity to learn what real people think. If things go well, a dialogue ensues, typically raising more questions, which can in turn form the basis of a further round of bundling, finding experts and reconvening.

Depending on the scale of the exercise, there may be more or fewer citizens, more or fewer questions, more or fewer experts, more or fewer rounds of dialogue.

The UK government has done this sort of thing a few times, as it happens, usually on difficult or contentious issues like genetic modification or nuclear power.[47] A cynical perspective might suggest that these were little more than elaborate market research exercises, since, if the 'answer' emerging from the process is not what had been hoped for by the government in question, little further action typically occurs.

But it's not only government that can do this sort of thing. The Joseph Rowntree Foundation has in recent years been calculating and publicizing a 'Minimum Income Standard' (MIS).[48] The MIS is 'based on what members of the public think is enough money to live on, to maintain a socially acceptable quality of life'. In essence, representatives of the general public – of the citizenry – go through a process to reach a consensus on what constitutes a 'socially acceptable quality of life'. There are no absolutes here. There is no right or wrong. It is entirely contextual, dependent on the prevailing norms – the prevailing stories – that society has. It is vernacular.

The citizens are supported through the process by experts such as sociologists and statisticians and even economists. The citizens don't actually work out the income – they focus on the goods and services that are implied by 'socially acceptable quality of life'. A television is included, for example – but it's the experts who trot off to find out how much it would cost, who tot up the costs of all the items included, and who work out what income would be necessary to fund such a lifestyle.

Even more directly relevant is the example of the Vincentian Partnership for Social Justice in Northern Ireland, which has not only calculated a Minimum Income Standard for Ireland but has established the cost of a 'healthy food basket'.[49] Using the same deliberative process, and bringing together ordinary citizens with expert nutritionists, they have established, firstly, what food items ought, for the purposes of a 'socially acceptable quality of life', to be in a weekly shopping basket; secondly, how much those items might cost in a variety of different situations; and, thirdly, what sort of income would be necessary to *afford* to eat healthily.

Which is to say: the process I am proposing for establishing what constitutes 'good', 'bad' and indifferent food already exists; it includes the views and perspectives of all segments of society, including the poor; and it works.

Of course, for the purposes of reconfiguring VAT as a twenty-first-century commitment device, a rather bigger exercise will be required. The Vincentian Partnership had sufficient resources to consider just two types of household and to work with relatively small groups of people from those household types. A national programme would require the participation of many hundreds of people, perhaps even thousands. It could easily take a couple of years. And it would cost many millions of pounds.*

But it would be a sum of money utterly dwarfed by our annual expenditure on tackling the obesity crisis. Prevention is not only better than the cure, it's cheaper too.

Step 2 of 4

I've assumed, for the moment and for the sake of simplicity, that the deliberative process of Step 1 has categorized food (and drink) into three groups: good, healthy items; unhealthy items; and everything else in the middle. There doesn't necessarily need to be three groups, but I'll return to that a little later.

For each group, it will be necessary to decide what the new VAT** rates should be. Like deciding which foods are healthy and which are not, this process is dauntingly difficult. How on earth can anyone know what sort of

---

* My business Brook Lyndhurst has practical insight into how big an exercise this might be. It may seem a task on the scale of Borges's Library of Babel to classify *every* food item; but beginning in 2009 and for several subsequent years, on behalf of WRAP and in order to collect authoritative data on food labelling and packaging, we catalogued more than 10,000 individual food items. And we learned, for example, just how much scope there is for consolidation: in a large supermarket there may, for example, be thirty different types of bread – but it's all bread.

** For simplicity's sake, I have retained the label 'VAT' throughout; in practice, I suspect that a new term or acronym may be required.

taxation rates will produce what kinds of changes in the amounts of healthy and unhealthy food that are bought? We saw earlier that the elasticities for individual products are very rarely known.

There are two parts to the answer. The first is to remember that this is not a once and once-only event; there will be opportunities in the years ahead to make adjustments – to change the rates, to change classifications, to change the number of bands. This process has its own established piece of jargon: test, learn, adapt. Once upon a time, when big government controlled big levers to make big things happen, it was possible to plan, devise and then put in place a huge and inflexible piece of infrastructure (levees, sewage systems, National Insurance) in order to tackle a social problem.

Such times are gone. Now we are in the era of diffused, complex problems, and they require new types of solution. Big complex systems are too big and too complex for anyone to devise a 'right' answer. The best way is to devise something at the level of principle and then test it, learn what worked and what didn't, and then adapt accordingly. Test, learn, adapt.

So if the bands aren't quite right, or the rates aren't quite right, no matter. Step 4 explains how we manage that.

But in the meantime, we still need to actually set the rates. And here, as with Step 1, we already have a model from which we can borrow.

Tax rates are presently set by the Chancellor of the Exchequer, which is to say that they are calculated by HM Treasury. This, remember, is one of the bastions wherein one finds the various priests and acolytes of the Theory. Putting that to one side, however, there is no doubting that there are some highly technical and difficult issues involved in setting tax rates (and this applies to income tax, too). There is therefore a good-looking case for saying that HM Treasury should be responsible for setting the new rates.

This solution would, however, fail to signal the new nature of the new VAT. HM Treasury's job is fiscal rectitude: to make sure, as far as possible, that the amount of money raised by government and the amount of money spent by government are roughly in line. It is not well positioned to deliver a new commitment device. Even if it were, the lack of public trust in government would be reason enough to reject this option: people simply wouldn't believe that the change was anything other than a money-raising exercise.

So the responsibility needs to reside elsewhere – an option that at first sight appears exceptionally challenging. But HM Treasury has been travelling along this path for some years already. Back in 1997 responsibility for setting interest rates was divested to the Monetary Policy Committee, specifically to 'de-politicize' this important tool of economic management. And in 2010 the government established the Office for Budget Responsibility, specifically to depoliticize the job of preparing economic forecasts.

While these examples demonstrate that HM Treasury can have no objection in principle to the idea of delegating responsibility elsewhere, neither example has either the structures or mechanisms to demonstrate fully the efficacy of the idea. That role falls to NICE – the National Institute for Health and Care Excellence. This is the body, originally set up in 1999, that (amongst other things) makes the decisions about which medicines are available through the NHS. Here is a task commensurate with the transformation of VAT. The NHS is the most cherished institution in Britain, and it affects every single citizen. Decisions on which medicines should be made available to which people are a very special kind of hard. The demand for health is virtually limitless, so there is a structural requirement to restrict (or ration) which health remedies – medicines, surgery, support and so forth – are available. In essence, life has to be priced, and different lives are unavoidably valued differently.

Not only that, but the players involved – national government, global pharmaceutical companies, health authorities, the general public, the mainstream media – are huge and powerful entities that scrutinize your every move and get very cross on a regular basis. And what did government do? Devolve responsibility so as to depoliticize the problem.

Here we have an arms-length entity that needs to remain trusted, or at least respected, by a broad and potentially very difficult group of constituents. An entity that is concerned with the nation's health, and huge sums of money. An entity that brings deep technical and professional expertise to bear so as to deliver against a set of objectives that has been set for it by a citizen-led process.

The new SmartVAT will require a hybrid of NICE and the Office for Budget Responsibility to administer the setting and monitoring of tax rates; and the success of these organizations gives us confidence that it can work.

To fail to give any idea of what sort of rates we might be talking about, however, would be to abrogate the responsibilities that come with putting forward a proposition such as this. So whilst it has to be the case that the *actual* rates would need to be set by the new NICE-like entity, my view is that the rate of VAT should be in the region of −20% on healthy foods, +25% on unhealthy foods, and +5% on everything else.

My thinking here is imprecise, and not just because I know it will be someone else's job to come up with the actual numbers. What is perhaps more important is test–learn–adapt: as I mentioned earlier, there are so many variables and so many unknowns all interacting in a fabulously complex system that *any* solution is going to need ongoing monitoring and refinement.*

---

* I have assumed that, certainly to begin with and for the purposes of these initial figures, it will be policy to ensure that the total tax take from the revised scheme is unchanged, i.e. that it is fiscally neutral.

So let's just focus on the healthy foods for a moment and ask ourselves whether a 20% reduction in the price of these foods will incentivize enough consumers to change their preferences (and, in turn, enough producers to switch or emerge to meet those preferences) sufficiently to have the hoped-for impact on obesity?* We don't know. It depends on the elasticity of demand for the food products in question; and on the relative shift compared with the now-more-expensive products; and how much consumer choices might have begun to shift in *advance* of the change in the expectation of its arrival. It also depends on something very slippery, which is that this thing we call price works in two separate ways: it is a formal, quantified and quantifiable thing that lends itself to precise calculation (if the item is £5 and you only have £4, you simply cannot buy it); but it is also symbolic, a signal, an indicator of something – which means it operates in the domain of narratives and stories and myths. The notion of a 'bargain' is the easiest illustration: simply knowing that the price of a thing is a 'bargain' invokes changes in whether or not you buy it, and how many you buy, irrespective of the actual price. (Another lovely example is the power of 99p or £99: everyone thinks they're immune to the oh-so-obvious ploy of charging £4.99 rather than £5,

---

* I envisage a process whereby the citizens and scientists of Step 1 and the NICE/OBR hybrid of Step 2 work together to agree the scale and timing of 'hoped for' effects.

or £499 rather than £500, but the reality is that, poor animal brains that we have, we fall for it almost all the time.[50] The symbol trumps the maths.)

And I have a hunch. I have a hunch that small percentage point differentials, which in pure economic terms might look big enough to shift our preferences, would not work. If the tax on healthy foods was, say, −2% and the tax on unhealthy foods was 5%, these would be differences not especially different from the kinds of variations in price with which consumers are already familiar. The signal being sent would simply be insufficient to prompt new choices. The commitment device would be too weak. My hunch is that a solid round number, −20%, sends a sufficiently strong signal *and* would produce a detectable difference on the receipt.

Turning to the unhealthy foods, the same logic applies. Twenty-five percent sounds like, and indeed is, a lot. But its most important feature is that it is slightly higher than the existing 'normal' VAT rate. The signal sent is that item X is not 'normal', it is unhealthy. Five percent tax on 'ordinary' foods is the same rate currently charged on domestic gas and electricity: it is conspicuously lower than the standard rate, but, in being a small positive figure, sends an important signal that it is different from the rate for healthy foods.

Step 3 of 4

The next step in the process is more practical. By this stage, remember, there are now three groups of food, each subject to a different rate of new VAT. It sounds like it might be an administrative nightmare.

The first part of the solution takes us back to my shopping trip in chapter 1. At no point in my day, whether I was buying chocolate or cigarettes or petrol or booze, was I informed at the point of purchase about the tax I was paying. This must change. Every food item on sale will have to clearly display the tax.* This may require some legislation; but, as for all the other elements discussed so far, the mechanisms either already exist or have been used elsewhere. Food products are legally obliged to convey nutritional information, for example; and their weight. Well, we're going to add 'tax' to the list.

I foresee that some retailers and manufacturers may wish to deploy some sort of ideogram or infographic to indicate which tax band each item belongs to. We have already seen traffic light indicators related to 'daily reference intake' (the even more incomprehensible successor to 'recommended daily allowance'). This is not acceptable. Whilst a green/amber/red mechanism could play a signalling role, it not only

---

* I do not address here the issue of the very small businesses that are not registered for VAT.

misses the other manifest aspect of price – its direct, quantitative character – but it also creates room for obfuscation.

This is of crucial importance for the negative tax rate. For the commitment device to be fully effective, consumers will need – I believe – to actually see the 'base' price, and then the negative tax, and then the final price. Whatever other offers may be put in place, by either the retailer or the producer, the price tag will show – for example – an original price of £1, a tax of –20p and a final price of 80p. It will very conspicuously look like a bargain: a 'money off' offer.

The second part of the solution to implementing a negative tax lies in the nature of an actual VAT return. I suspect that not very many people have ever actually completed a VAT return; but I have. Many times. As the owner–manager of a small enterprise, it was my joy once a quarter to complete the form. The business eventually reached a size whereby we could employ someone specifically to fill it in for me, but even then I had to check and sign it.

The single most important thing to know is that you do not have to tell Her Majesty's Revenue & Customs (the HMRC: the people who collect tax on behalf of government) which items you sold. If you sold fifty boxes of biscuits, you don't at any point have to say 'I sold fifty boxes of biscuits'. Or, if you sell both biscuits and crisps, you don't have to tell them that, either. What you have to do is tell them the total value of goods sold at any particular VAT rate; and, then, how much VAT you collected.

So if you're a big supermarket and you're selling tens of thousands of items during the course of a week, you will need to do four sums under this new regime. First, what was the total value of the items you sold that were subject to the −20% tax? Second, what was the value of the items at +5%? Third, the total of those at +25%. And fourth, add them up.

So, just to make this completely clear, let's look at the following table.

Category	Net value of sales (£)	VAT (£)
Healthy food (−20%)	10,000	−2,000
Normal food (+5%)	10,000	+500
Unhealthy food (+25%)	10,000	+2,500
Total	30,000	+1,000

The retailer puts these numbers into the VAT return (it's electronic these days, of course) and pays HMRC £1,000. Simple as.

And, whilst this might once have been a genuine administrative nightmare (it certainly would have been in the years when I was stacking shelves in a supermarket: each item was priced with a sticky piece of paper, and it was only the price that was registered at the till), it is absolutely not the case now. Every single item is barcoded.

And this is the third and final part of how negative VAT can work, and how the actual administrative burden on retailers will be marginal. I predict that they won't like being obliged to make clear to consumers how much tax they are or are not paying; but calculating the VAT is something that will require no more than a once-only investment of a few hours of coding.

Step 4 of 4

So there we have it. A transparent and inclusive and well-funded deliberative process, involving both citizens and scientists, to allocate foods to one of three bundles. An entity at arm's length from government and/or HM Treasury – a sort of hybrid between the Office for Budget Responsibility and the National Institute for Health and Care Excellence – to set the tax rates. And retailers, obliged to display the tax rates in monetary terms, and obliged as they already are to add up some numbers and fill in a form once a quarter.

The remaining issue is, as I said earlier, that the whole thing will be imperfect. No amount of thought or research or design beforehand will be able to eliminate this virtual certainty. It is in the nature of complex systems. The solution is: test, learn, adapt.

So the final step is to have a mechanism for monitoring how it all works, and adjusting it as we go along. It would probably not be a good idea to be making *continuous* adjustments, either to which foods go in which category or to what rates are charged; that really would be a headache. But a review with an annual or biennial or even triennial cycle would seem reasonable. Again, the precedent and mechanisms already exist: the bundle of items used by the Office for National Statistics to calculate retail price inflation is updated on an annual basis, with some now-less-popular items leaving the list and new now-more-popular items joining each year. It would be straightforward to mimic this for the new VAT.

Or it could be aligned with the Comprehensive Spending Review, which runs on a three-year cycle.

If we discover that you, I and millions of other people responded more dramatically than we anticipated, we can revise down the rates. If we discover that particular food groups respond more or less quickly compared with our expectations, we may move them into another tax band. If total tax revenue falls more than expected, we can have a rethink. We test the original design by monitoring it carefully and continuously; we learn, in an open and transparent and grown-up fashion (we don't pretend it's someone's 'fault' and start hiding or blaming); and we adapt it, in light of what we learn.

Chapter 10

Not everyone will be happy

> Without leaps of imagination or dreaming, we lose the excitement of possibilities. Dreaming, after all, is a form of planning.
>
> — *Gloria Steinem*

B ut could SmartVAT be implemented, really? And if it was put in place, would it really work?

As to the first question, I'm doubtful. The resistance will be considerable, perhaps overwhelming. The economists would claim that it's too much of a distortion to the market – despite the fact that SmartVAT would be a more transparent and rational distortion than the taxes it would replace.

The Treasury would argue that it would be fabulously expensive and would risk reducing the amount of revenue government receives – despite the fact that it would be dramatically less expensive than continuing to meet the costs of obesity, that it could just as easily increase revenue, and that it has a self-correcting mechanism built in.

A government of any hue would consider the political risks to be too high, despite the use of third-party institutions of a kind with which it is already comfortable. And the media would simply cleave along established political lines, identifying one group or another for whom the change would be profoundly unfair.

The media reaction would also, of course, be informed by the commercial interests that lie behind it; and there seems little doubt that the reaction of the large retailers and food manufacturers would be powerfully hostile. This proposal is, after all, based on a proposition that these businesses have been systematically benefiting from a profound asymmetry. Redressing the asymmetry would certainly lead to, at a minimum, a realignment of the corporate landscape.

It's curious, though, that such realignments are so often bitterly resisted, then smoothly accepted once they're in place. Businesses often call for a 'level playing field', this being no more than a request that the rules apply equally to everyone. On that playing field, so long as it's level, businesses can compete with one another to do whatever it is they do. That, surely, is the Darwinian way. SmartVAT is no more than a change in the rules, a change in the shape or nature of the playing field. The smart, innovative, agile businesses will adapt and thrive; the monolithic will struggle and fail. What's new there? Perhaps there would be shop closures or job losses or reduced investment – as there would be new types of provision, new jobs and new types of investment. What's new there?

Perhaps the biggest resistance to the change, however, would come from us – from consumers themselves. Increase the price of my favourite cake/chocolate/ready meal? You must be joking – that just isn't fair! And what about poor people (we'll say)? They're bound to suffer disproportionately if you make food more expensive.

But the system is already unfair. It's been unfair for so long that we barely notice anymore. Cheap, convenient food is unfair – not just on the animals that lead horrific lives away from our gaze, or on the workers that have to survive on pitiful wages out of our sight, or on the planetary environment as it suffers beyond our horizons. It's unfair because it exploits the illusion of choice, in the interests of capital, to jeopardize the future health of millions of people. And it is not, in general, the prosperous middle classes who are getting fat – it is the poor, the disadvantaged, the less well educated, the people who already have the least choice in their lives as a result of the jobs that they do and the incomes that they have.

SmartVAT is a way of redressing the unfairness. It doesn't simply make some foods more expensive, it makes many foods more affordable. It has, as a prize, better health. Properly designed – which means making sure that the interests of all groups of society are taken into account when deciding what counts as healthy and what counts as unhealthy food – it has the potential to have a dramatic positive effect on something that most people think is the most important thing there is.

Which is my answer to the second question with which I began this chapter. Would it work? Yes.

Not only that, SmartVAT invites us to think about our other bad habits, and it hints at ways in which we might commit to profoundly better choices.

Chapter 11

New choices and new possibilities

> [By 2056] Darwinian critiques of consumer capitalism should undermine the social and sexual appeal of conspicuous consumption. Absurdly wasteful display will become less popular once people comprehend its origins in sexual selection, and its pathetic unreliability as a signal of individual merit or value.
>
> — Dr Geoffrey Miller

I mentioned earlier that climate change has been described as the 'mother of all externalities'. That is, it is the biggest cost imposed by business that is not paid by business and is thus not included in the price we pay for things. It's not 'just' business, of course. I said, too, that Western lifestyles were largely to blame: the energy and resources needed to support our Western lifestyles are out of all kilter with the ability of the planet either to supply the raw materials or absorb all the waste products (including carbon dioxide) that such lifestyles imply.

You know this already, of course. We are all familiar with the idea that we need three planets to support our lifestyles and we have (at the last count) just one available.[51]

Eventually we (in its very widest sense) are going to need a very different kind of economy, one that really is consistent with a finite planet. Many – and I am one – call this a 'sustainable economy'. Some – and again I am one – take this to mean not only an economy that is environmentally sustainable, but one that is socially just, too. In fact, my preferred way of characterizing a 'sustainable economy' is one that inverts the current model completely: at present, we inhabit an economy where the needs of 'the economy' seem to come first, and everything else – you, me, our communities and cultures, the very planet as a whole – must bend to meet its needs. A sustainable economy, for me, is one in which our needs come first – the need for health, the need for conviviality, the need for a healthy planet – and this thing we call an economy is configured to meet those needs.

I am of the view that a sustainable economy can and will come about only when we want one. There are only two sides in an economy: supply and demand. So far, almost all of the effort to bring about a more sustainable economy (for which read a green or resource-efficient or circular economy) has focused on the supply side. That is, it has focused on the processes by which the things we buy are made and it has tried to make them less harmful. Let's use less energy while making all these things; let's use fewer hazardous chemicals; let's try to reduce the amount of waste in the supply chain; and so on.

These supply-side efforts are, sadly, inevitably and ceaselessly dwarfed by the combined effects of the requirements of capital and the desires of consumers. Capital – disembodied, seemingly no longer under anyone's control and called 'the markets' – is relentless in its quest for a return, and it has at its disposal the most sophisticated means of engineering our consent through the construction of powerful stories and myths. Capital is entirely comfortable with notions such as 'resource efficiency' because it translates directly into notions such as 'lower operating costs'. These, in turn, translate directly into the profits that capital requires. Even the more sophisticated models in which consumers no longer 'own' things but merely lease them offer only marginal resistance to the overall direction of travel.

We, comprehensively suffused by the powerful and sophisticated myths required to maintain the returns that capital requires, keep wanting more televisions, more home furnishings, more exotic foods, more holidays – all using up finite resources far faster than any efficiency gains can hope to balance out.

If we really did make more sustainable choices – well, businesses would supply them. That's what the supply side does. If there's demand out there, someone somewhere will figure out a way to supply it. Isn't that (part of) what capitalism is about?

There are those that think we can rely on 'behaviour change' to get us there. The argument runs something like this: if we can persuade people to recycle, and use water more sparingly, and buy locally grown food, and use less electricity, and use less gas, and drive less frequently, then these things will come together to produce a change in mindset, a shift in how consumers think, and therefore behave, towards 'sustainable'.

There are others that believe a deeper shift in values is required. Rather than expressing ourselves through 'extrinsic' means, runs this argument, we instead need to express ourselves through 'intrinsic' values. Rather than buy for ourselves (extrinsic) we need to care for others (intrinsic). Rather than seek affirmation through display, we need to foster our internal wisdom. Rather than shop, we should sing.[52]

I myself have conducted plenty of research in recent years on environmental behaviour change;[53] and, by and large, I think it's a good thing. Sometimes it even works. Take the case of food waste, for example: the UK leads the world in tackling food waste by consumers, almost entirely on the basis of a sustained behaviour-change campaign by WRAP.[54] Or the case of Change4Life, a successful programme to promote healthier lifestyles from the Department of Health and aimed at key vulnerable groups.[55] (If you don't know about it, that's because it's not aimed at you.)

And I have a lot of sympathy, too, with arguments about values. A world in which the majority of people were acting on the basis of intrinsic rather than extrinsic values would indeed be more sustainable.

But neither of these approaches is anywhere near powerful enough to redress the asymmetry I've been describing; and progress over the past decade or so has been far too slow to make any serious difference. If we are serious – and by that I mean something like 'if we seriously want to avoid a genuine global catastrophe' – we need to move much more directly and much more quickly.

SmartVAT gives a hint of what might be required, and in and of itself would provide a powerful kick to the process of positive change. There is no inevitable or preordained destination to which this thing we call an economy is heading – it really is ours. It really is us. If we want to make it grow and evolve in a new direction, we can make that happen: we need merely the commitment to formulate the necessary commitment devices. Once it starts evolving in a new direction, the same organic processes that kept it going in the direction it's been going for the past sixty or seventy years would keep it going in the new direction. Darwinian evolution may have produced the red-in-tooth-and-claw selfishness so often used to characterize the essential nature of capitalism, but it also produced the ability to care and collaborate upon which we also manifestly depend.

I've sketched out a mechanism for using the price mechanism to tackle obesity – but it could, in principle, go much further than that. There is no reason, for example, why the bands into which the various food stuffs are allocated should be restricted simply to 'healthy' and 'unhealthy'; they could be further subdivided with respect to environmental issues. Good for you and good for the planet – high negative SmartVAT; bad for you and bad for the planet – higher positive SmartVAT; and so on.

One could add in income inequalities: bad for you, bad for the planet and only bought by really wealthy people – very high SmartVAT. Et cetera. You get the idea.

We know we can't carry blithely on. Deep down, we don't really want to destroy the planet; we don't really want our fellow humans to suffer the indignities of injustice; we don't really want to be fat. As citizens, in calm repose, we can sincerely wish that, from tomorrow onwards, we don't eat so much rubbish. In this book, I've shown how we could construct and put in place a commitment strategy to help us do just that. It's a strategy that's open, transparent, accountable, adaptable, inclusive and built up from component parts that have all been shown to work in other settings.

Box 5 shows the results of a couple of survey questions I asked, one a decade or so ago, one more recently. I asked a representative sample of the British public

Box 5

In 2003 Brook Lyndhurst commissioned MORI to conduct a survey with a representative sample (n = 1,013) of the British public, asking the following question.

'How fair do you think it would be if the government were to introduce a lower rate of VAT on energy efficient light-bulbs and a higher rate of VAT on normal lightbulbs?'

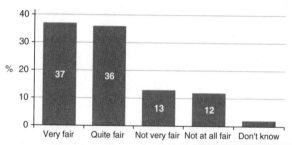

In 2013, a decade later, we updated the question a little and GfK asked the following on our behalf.

'How fair do you think it would be if the government were to introduce a lower rate of VAT on energy efficient prod-ucts and a higher rate of VAT on normal products?'

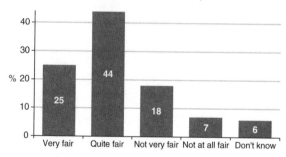

whether they thought it would be *fair* or *unfair* if government were to reduce the price of an environmentally good option whilst simultaneously increasing the price of an environmentally harmful option. I asked about electrical items rather than food, but the pattern is dramatically clear and would I'm sure be replicated with food: the overwhelming majority of us think it would be fair to make the 'good' choices cheaper and the 'bad' choices more expensive.

I think this is the best thing about SmartVAT: it would be fair. It would redress a long-standing and unfair imbalance in the kinds of choices we really have; and it could make sure that those in our society that invariably bear the brunt of life are considered and protected.

I think it would be fair; and so, I believe, would millions of other people.

Endnotes

1. GOV.UK. 2015. Tax on shopping and services. At www.gov.uk/tax -on-shopping (accessed 29 October 2015).

2. HM Revenue and Customs. 2015. HMRC tax and NIC receipts: monthly and annual historical record. At www.gov.uk/government/ uploads/system/uploads/attachment_data/file/468810/Sep15_Recei pts_NS_Bulletin_Final.pdf (accessed 29 October 2015).

3. All taxation figures in this section are accurate as of October 2015.

4. See endnote 2. Government receipts from taxing tobacco were equivalent to around 0.5% of GDP in 2014–15: roughly three times larger than all environmental taxes combined.

5. House of Commons Library. 2015. Alcohol: minimum pricing. Briefing Paper 5021. At http://researchbriefings.parliament.uk/Rese archBriefing/Summary/SN05021 (accessed 29 October 2015).

6. See p. 14 of endnote 2. The escalator was introduced in 1993 and abandoned in 2000.

7. R. Thaler and C. Sunstein. 2008. *Nudge: Improving Decisions about Health, Wealth and Happiness*. New Haven, CT: Yale University Press. See also Defra/Brook Lyndhurst. 2006. Nudging the S-curve. At http://randd.defra.gov.uk/Default.aspx?Menu=Menu&Module= More&Location=None&Completed=0&ProjectID=13990 (accessed 29 October 2015).

8. E. Johnson and D. Goldstein. 2003. Do defaults save lives? *Science* 302:1338–1339. At www.dangoldstein.com/papers/DefaultsScience .pdf (accessed 29 October 2015).

9. S. Mullainathan and E. Shafir. 2013. *Scarcity: Why Having Too Little Means So Much*. New York: Time Books.

10. N. Mammarella, B. Fairfield, A. Di Domenico and T. Di Fiore. 2013. Baby on board: reducing risk taking in adult drivers in a simulated driving game. *Accident Analysis & Prevention* 50:596–599. At www.sciencedirect.com/science/article/pii/S0001457512003405 (accessed 29 October 2015).

11. L. Moutinho, ed. 2014. *The Routledge Companion to the Future of Marketing*. London: Taylor & Francis.

12. M. Moss. 2013. *Salt, Sugar, Fat: How the Food Giants Hooked Us*. New York: Penguin Random House.

13. R. Wilkinson and K. Pickett. 2009. *The Spirit Level: Why More Equal Societies Almost Always Do Better*. London: Allen Lane.

14. UCL. 2013. How 'obesity gene' triggers weight gain. At www.ucl.ac.uk/news/news-articles/0713/15072013-How-obesity-gene-triggers-weight-gain-Batterham (accessed 8 November 2015).

15. C. Wallis. 2014. How gut bacteria make us fat and thin. *Scientific American*. At www.scientificamerican.com/article/how-gut-bacteria-help-make-us-fat-and-thin/ (accessed 8 November 2015).

16. H. Walton et al. 2015. *Understanding the Health Impacts of Air Pollution in London*. London: King's College London/Greater London Authority.

17. R. Tol. 2012. The economic effects of climate change. *Journal of Economic Perspectives* 23(2):29–51.

18. K. Armstrong. 2005. *A Short History of Myth*. London: Canongate.

19. D. Dennett. 1995. *Darwin's Dangerous Idea*. London: Simon & Schuster.

20. E. Canetti. 1960. *Crowds and Power*. London: Gollanz.

21. T. Veblen. 1899. *The Theory of the Leisure Class: An Economic Study in the Evolution of Institutions*. New York: B. W. Huebsch.

22. F. Hirsch. 1976. *The Social Limits to Growth*. Henley-on-Thames: Routledge & Kegan Paul.

23. J. Keynes. 1930. Economic possibilities for our grandchildren. In *Essays in Persuasion* (J. Keynes, 1963). New York: W.W. Norton & Co.

24. Age UK. 2015. Walk your way to health. At www.ageuk.org.uk/health-wellbeing/keeping-fit/walk-your-way-to-health/how-walking-can-improve-your-health/ (accessed 8 November 2015).

25. F. Gros. 2014. *A Philosophy of Walking*. London: Verso.

26. Brook Lyndhurst. 2010. Social capital: a rural perspective. Project undertaken for Defra.

27. NHS Choices. 2014. Walking for health. At www.nhs.uk/Livewell/getting-started-guides/Pages/getting-started-walking.aspx (accessed 8 November 2015).

28. Office for National Statistics. 2013. Measuring national well-being: what matters most to personal well-being? At www.ons.gov.uk/ons/rel/wellbeing/measuring-national-well-being/what-matters-most-to-personal-well-being-in-the-uk-/art-what-matters-most-to-personal-well-being-in-the-uk-.html#tab-abstract (accessed 8 November 2015).

29. GOV.UK. 2011. People want to buy healthy, local food, survey shows. At www.gov.uk/government/news/people-want-to-buy-healthy-local-food-survey-shows (accessed 8 November 2015).

30. Brook Lyndhurst. 2010. Are labels the answer? Barriers to buying higher welfare products. Project undertaken for Defra.

31. R. Dunbar. 1998. The social brain hypothesis. *Evolutionary Anthropology* 6:178–190.

32. G. Lakoff and M. Johnson. 1980. *Metaphors We Live By*. University of Chicago Press.

33. D. Miller. 1998. *A Theory of Shopping*. London: Wiley.

34. A. Offer. 2007. *The Challenge of Affluence: Self-Control and Well-Being in the United States and Britain Since 1950*. Oxford University Press.

35. T. Schelling. 2007. *Strategies of Commitment and Other Essays*. Cambridge, MA: Harvard University Press.

36. Action on Smoking and Health (ASH). 2015. Tobacco industry. At www.ash.org.uk/information/tobacco-industry (accessed 8 November 2015).

37. British Medical Association. 2015. *Food for Thought: Promoting Healthy Diets among Children and Young People*. London: BMA.

38. GOV.UK. 2013. Salt strategy aims to reduce our salt consumption by a quarter. At www.gov.uk/government/news/salt-strategy-aims -to-help-reduce-our-salt-consumption-by-a-quarter (accessed 8 November 2015).

39. NHS. 2015. Change4Life. At www.nhs.uk/change4life/Pages/cha nge-for-life.aspx (accessed 8 November 2015).

40. S. Smed. 2012. Financial penalties on foods: the fat tax in Denmark. *Nutrition Bulletin* 37:142–147.

41. Public Health England. 2015. *Sugar Reduction: The Evidence for Action*. London: PHE.

42. Scottish Government. 2015. Minimum pricing. At www.gov.scot/ Topics/Health/Services/Alcohol/minimum-pricing (accessed 8 November 2015).

43. OECD. 2015. Trust in government. At www.oecd.org/gov/trust -in-government.htm (accessed 8 November 2015).

44. J. Nickerson and R. Sanders. 2014. *Tackling Wicked Government Problems*. Washington DC: Brookings Institution Press.

45. Stanford University. 2015. Centre for Deliberative Democracy. At http://cdd.stanford.edu/ (accessed 8 November 2015).

46. K. Roberts and K. Marvin. 2011. Knowledge and attitudes towards healthy eating and physical activity: what the data tell us. Report, National Obesity Observatory, Oxford.

47. Department for Business, Enterprise & Regulatory Reform. 2008. Meeting the energy challenge: a white paper on nuclear power. HMSO, London.

48. Joseph Rowntree Foundation. 2015. Minimum income standards. At www.jrf.org.uk/topic/mis (accessed 25 November 2015).

49. Food Standards Agency. 2015. Cost of a healthy food basket for households on the island of Ireland. At www.food.gov.uk/science/ research/devolvedadmins/fs411025 (accessed 25 November 2015).

50. N. Lacetera, D. Pope and J. Syndor. 2011. Heuristic thinking and limited attention in the car market. Paper 17030, National Bureau of Economic Research.

51. Bioregional. 2015. One planet living. At www.bioregional.com/oneplanetliving/ (accessed 25 November 2015).

52. D. Fell. 2013. Let's sing, not shop: an economist dreams of a sustainable city. In *Imagining the Future City: London 2062* (ed. S. Bell and J. Paskins). London: Ubiquity Press.

53. Brook Lyndhurst. 2015. Behaviour change, lifestyles and well-being. At www.brooklyndhurst.co.uk/behaviour-change-lifestyles-and-wellbeing-_19 (accessed 25 November 2015).

54. Wrap. 2015. Love food, hate waste. At www.lovefoodhatewaste.com/ (accessed 25 November 2015).

55. NHS Choices. 2015. Change4Life. At www.nhs.uk/change4life/Pages/change-for-life.aspx (accessed 25 November 2015).